How To Top Like A Stud

A Penetrating Guide To Gay Sex

By Woody Miller

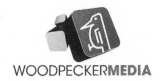

WOODPECKER**MEDIA**

Table Of Contents

How To Stop Worrying That Your Penis Isn't Big Enough.

Journal Of Sex Medicine Survey: Penis Size Stats For White, Black & Hispanic Men

Introduction

I've been writing about gay sex for over ten years. I starred in an international hit TV show called The Sex Inspectors (it aired in 12 countries, including the U.S. (HBO) and the U.K. (Channel Four). I've answered thousands of questions over the course of my career, interviewed dozens of sexologists and read hundreds of books, articles, columns, surveys and research papers on gay sex. And you know what? I've almost never seen an article, let alone a book on how to penetrate men. There are a lot of books on bottoming but topping? None. Zero. Zilch. Why?

A reader to my sex advice column once wrote me this:

I always hear guys saying, "I love it when a top knows what to do." But they never specify just what that top is doing that is so great! I know there's the whole massaging of the prostate thing, but if you're a top can you really feel the prostate that well with your dick? I mean, let's get super specific here guys and let me know exactly what a great top does. Is it a certain fuck stroke, is it just being patient with you, is it more psychological things he does like acting dominant? What the hell makes a great top?

My sentiments exactly. What makes a great top? And back to the point I made earlier, why is the information so hard to come by? Partly it's because men do not like to admit ignorance on a topic they're supposed to know about. Partly

3

it's because there's a perception that there's not much to topping—get it hard, put it in, end of story. If you watch porn (and who doesn't?) you know there is no such thing as a top wondering what to do. The performer gets hard and sticks it in. No ifs, ands or buts. Actually, there are a lot of butts, but I digress.

Perhaps the biggest reason for the paucity of information on topping is that unlike bottoming, there is no pain associated with it. And pain avoidance is a motivating force for learning an activity. There is a LOT of pain associated with bottoming if you don't know what you're doing. And because there is, lots of people write about it and lots more read about it.

But topping? Not so much. While there is no physical pain associated with topping (unless your partner is tighter than a jar of glue) there is often a lot of confusion, awkwardness and sexual dissatisfaction.

What if the "yuck factor"—the smell or unsightly stains that can accompany anal sex—ruins your erection? A lot of men want to top other guys but they can't get past the visual and olfactory obstacles. What are they to do?

And what about the guys who have performance anxiety? There you are, rock hard until the moment of penetration. Then suddenly Willie becomes Will Not. How do you get around the psychological obstacles to being a penetrator?

And of course, there's everyone's favorite—condom-causing impotence. There you are, rock hard (what is it with you and rocks?), but when the condom comes on and you suddenly feel like you're trying to play pool with a rope. How do you solve that riddle?

The problems don't end there. What if you're dealing with a newbie who's never bottomed before or is simply not very experienced. What should you do or say to make him comfortable? Telling him to "Relax! Relax!" is actually the worst thing you could say to him. You know how irritated you feel when you're at a bar and a friend says, "Smile! Smile!" You want to punch him. Same thing with your partner. He's not going to appreciate a glib "relax!" while you try to insert a pole that is 10x the size of his orifice.

Getting your penis in poses a few tactical challenges. What's the best angle of entry? What's the best position to start with? How are your knees holding up? How do you keep hard while you're trying to figure it out?

And once you're in you're tasked with doing double duty—giving as well as taking pleasure. Do you "make love" or give him a back alley pounding? Do you go soft and gentle or fuck like a runaway jackhammer? There are actually thrusting patterns that men who bottom enjoy more than others. I bet nobody ever told you about that, huh? Well, until now.

And finally, there's the issue of premature ejaculation. It

isn't unusual for men who top to ejaculate way before they want to. As you will soon see, a good top does not 'finish' until his partner does.

Whew! That's a lot of issues for the simple act of topping. Wasn't it supposed to be easy as (warm) pie? Well, if it were that easy then we'd all be having anal intercourse, wouldn't we? Sadly, gay men have a lot less anal sex than you'd think. The Journal Of Sex Medicine shocked the gay community a while back with its sex survey of 25,000 gay men in all 50 states. It asked a simple question: "Have you engaged in anal sex in the past month?" Guess how many guys said yes?

Thirty-seven percent!

That wasn't a typo. Thirty seven percent! And yet, all you hear about is whether somebody's a top, bottom or versatile. It's in our app profiles, our jokes (*"Why did the gay man cross the road? He heard the chicken was a top"*) and our insults (*"There's nothing but bottoms in this town"*).

Clearly, anal sex isn't that easy for a lot of gay men. Bottoming gets the nod for the most problematic act but the Journal of Sex Medicine's survey results hints at a more silent one—the obstacles associated with topping. Most of us have some level of apprehension associated with the issues I've just outlined (from cleanliness to tightness), and until now, there's been very little we could read about that could help us work through it.

My intention is to help you blast through the issues that prevent you from topping successfully. Whether you're new to the scene, are exclusively bottom-oriented and want to be more versatile, or you're an exclusively top-oriented guy but want to be better at it—you're going to find stellar advice to maximize your pleasure.

You ready to start? Then get your hands out of your pants and turn the page. Let's get to work!

CHAPTER ONE

Discovering Your Inner Top

*How To Express The Kind Of Masculinity
You Feel Comfortable With*

Topping somebody isn't just about inserting your penis into his orifice. If it were strictly a physical sensation you could accomplish the same thing with a dildo. No, topping is way more than the physical act of inserting your penis. It's a constellation of masculine expressions that orbit around one word: Domination.

Now, domination is a loaded word. It's exciting for people who are clear about what they like—total tops who want to express it or total bottoms who want to submit to it. But it's also a scary word for would-be tops because it has the connotation that only "real men"—macho men, tall men, big men, hung men have the right to top. Not only that, but the word 'domination' also conjures up whips, chains, slings, dimly lit basements and the darker side of the psyche.

So, where does THAT definition of domination leave you if you're not a hyper masculine man who just wants to be a more versatile lover?

A lot of guys won't entertain the idea of topping because they feel they have to step into a role they're not comfortable in. If you think the only way you can pleasure your partner is to "act" with the kind of hyper-masculinity that makes you uncomfortable, then it's easy to see why you'd stay away from topping.

Let's talk about roles for a minute because this is a huge stumbling block for a lot of gay men. Let's delve into the negative stereotypes associated with bottoming and then flip it around to see how a kind of reverse stereotype stops many men from topping.

In ancient Greece and Rome being the penetrator was synonymous with being a man. Anything that subverted the concept of masculinity was punished with social ostracism and ridicule. And nothing mocked masculinity more than getting penetrated.

Greeks and Romans didn't really care whom you had sex with (women, men, boys, slaves) as long as you were the penetrator. The Romans even had a word for it: *Vir.* It was an exalted term, symbolizing the ideal man: He who penetrates other men but is himself not penetrated.

Today we still live out those vestiges of antiquity. We label men "tops" or "bottoms" in part because we're living out antiquity's fear of the feminine. In heterosexual thinking, the penetrator (man) is more valuable than the penetrated (women). We've adapted that consciousness in our own community, where the penetrator (top) is more valuable than the penetrated (bottom).

Clearly, labels like "top" and "bottom" can be useful shorthand for sexual likes and dislikes. But instead of stating what we prefer—"I like to bottom"—we turned that preference into an identity—"I'm a bottom."

By developing identities out of these labels we cut ourselves off of any unlabeled possibilities. In our world, tops can only date or hook up with bottoms and bottoms can only do the same with tops. That's a whole lot of blindness in a sighted community.

I Call Bullshit.

To say that topping is more masculine than bottoming is nonsense. Just like your sexual orientation says nothing about your character, your preference for topping over bottoming says nothing about your masculinity.

Labels Belong On Can, Not A Man.

I don't like the words "top", "bottom" or even "versatile" because in the end, they're labels. And while labels can sometimes act as helpful linguistic shorthand, they almost always morph into psychic prisons preventing you from experiencing all that there is to experience.

There is no shame in being gay; there is no shame in liking

to receive. Conversely, there is no pride in topping. The only thing shameful is how willing we are to buy into such bogus identities. You will note throughout this book that I rarely use the words "top" or "bottom" as identities, only as verbs. I do not think you are a "top" because you prefer to insert. I do not think you are a "bottom" because you like to receive. Unless you can start seeing these words as verbs instead of identities, it will be difficult for you to mentally relax enough to take either role with zest and pleasure.

How Labels Stop Guys From Bottoming.

Your conscious mind will be so fearful of losing its perceived sense of masculinity that you start thinking things like, "If I bottom it means deep down that I'm a woman." Your subconscious will protect you from that unthinkable thought by making your sphincter so tight no amount of relaxation exercises will loosen you up.

The Journal of Sex Medicine's survey showed that only 37% of gay men reported having anal sex in the previous month. Clearly, the obstacles to topping contribute to this low figure.

How Labels Stop Guys From Topping.

Your conscious mind will be so fearful of an inability to pull off a testosterone-laden caveman macho prick act that you start thinking things like "I'm not mean enough—or hung enough—to be a top." Your subconscious will support that thought by making you impotent until you're at a safe enough distance from the role you mistakenly think you have to play.

As you can see, there are plenty of emotional blocks that can stop men from either topping or bottoming. And surely that contributes to the dismayingly low rates of consensual anal sex between gay men discovered by the Journal Of Sex Medicine's survey (only 37% of gay men reported having anal sex in the previous month).

If you're having trouble accessing your inner top, it's because you have a limiting view of masculinity. You have a list of "shoulds" that keep you from pleasurably experiencing what it's like to be the 'active' participant in a coupling. That list includes but is not limited to thoughts like:

- I'm not tall enough

- I don't weigh enough

- My voice isn't deep enough

- My dick isn't big enough

- I'm not aggressive enough

- I'm not built well enough

- I'm not man enough

- I wear caftans for Chrissakes!

If you recognize yourself in these statements you've bought into a big lie. You've limited yourself to playing in a tiny puddle when a vast unexplored ocean beckons. The idea that only hung macho pricks should top is about as valid as saying that only effeminate men should bottom. Buying into either assumption locks you into a psychic prison that keep you from experiencing new levels of sexual joy and satisfaction.

The Top Whisperer.
It's one thing to understand a problem; it's another to solve it. If at this point you've come to the realization that you've indeed bought into the toxic role-playing assumptions listed above, what can you actually do about it?

For one, you can start saying what some backwoods southerners like to say when they've come up against something they don't like: *"Devil, I refute thee!!"* In other words, consciously refute your assumptions. For example, this idea that you can only top if your dick is so big you need Dropbox to send dic pics? Call it out. It simply isn't true. Condom companies say that only 6% of the population needs an extra-large condom. How can you hear a statistic like that without putting a dent into the false belief that tops should be hung? That means only 6% of the population gets to top? I think not.

And size queens aside, most guys who bottom would MUCH rather do it for an average-sized guy than a guy whose dick is so big it's in the next room mixing drinks. My point is that facts have a destabilizing influence on false assumptions. Use them often enough and your assumptions will start to crumble.

Being A Top Doesn't Mean Acting Like A Cop.

There are two basic assumptions that can keep a guy from topping. We've talked about the first—that you 'should' be tall, muscled, hung or whatever your tightly defined stereotype is for masculinity. The second is what you should do— dominate aggressively and be physically rough and forceful. One 'should' springs from the other. All you're allowed to be determines all you're allowed to do. If all you're allowed to be is a Dom top then all you're allowed to do is Dom-ish things. Like being forceful, rough, selfish and the rest of the negative connotations that come from a singular view of what domination means.

The idea that domination has to take a certain form is yet another 'should' that needs to be taken out to the woodshed and spanked. There is no question that being a top requires you to take on a more masculine role. That is beyond contention. What is up for debate and what can help you overcome the limiting notion of an out of reach masculinity, is how you approach that active role.

The Submissive Top.

You can top someone without taking on the kind of mascu-

> The idea that only hung macho pricks should top is about as valid as saying that only effeminate men should bottom. Both lock you into a psychic prison.

linity you feel uncomfortable with. You can top someone without pretending to be something you're not. You can completely enjoy the active role without descending into stereotypes. There are many ways of expressing domination. You can do it tenderly and you can do it roughly. And you can do it in various degrees of both. One is not better than the other. It all depends on what you're comfortable with and what your partner wants.

It is even possible to top submissively. If you've ever seen a power bottom at work you will see that the top is pretty much playing the submissive role. Yes, it is his penis doing the penetrating but it's the bottom completely controlling everything—from the depth and speed of the thrusts to what positions they take and for how long.

Again, there is no one way to be a top and there is no one way of expressing "topulinity" if I may coin a term.

Embrace The Power Without Giving Up Your Identity.
Let's talk about power for a moment because it is central to your success as a top. As I've said before, power is expressed in many different forms. Everyone who has sex plays

with some degree of power whether they acknowledge it or not. You are either exerting it or submitting to it in everything from kissing to mutual masturbation to oral sex and of course, anal sex.

ALL people play with power. It's just that few of us ever label it that way. Let's take something as innocent as kissing. If you like to be pinned under your guy when you're kissing, you've experienced the thrill of submitting to power. If you like being on top of him while you kiss, you've experienced the thrill of wielding it. It's not possible to have any act of romance or sex without some kind of power exchange. At one moment or another you are wielding or yielding.

If you're doing missionary, you are surrendering yourself to him. If you're on top guiding the speed and depth of his thrusts, you're controlling him. If you dig your nails into his back, you've inflicted pain. If he does it, you've had pain inflicted on you. If you've liked a massage that almost hurts, you've experienced a pleasurable aspect of pain. If you've given one, you've experienced the satisfaction of administering it.

Just because you're not conscious of how you relate to and enjoy power doesn't mean you're not experiencing it. But starting today you can come at it with awareness and intent. You can become aware of the kind of power you're attracted to and create the environment for a satisfying experience. In a moment I'm going to help you with an organized, systematic attempt at understanding the power sensations you're drawn to. For now, let's explore the dynamics of sexual intercourse.

Topping and bottoming require a consensual exchange of power. You can be submissive (choosing to allow the other person to have control over you in some way) or dominant (choosing to honor the request). Notice the words "choose" and "allow." They are critical to consensual, structured power playing.

Any relationship to power holds its own individual thrill. Submitting to power, for example, often elicits an exhilarating, liberating feeling. By giving up responsibility for what's going on, by bending your will to the authority of another, by taking on the role of the compliant receiver, you can experience a form of therapeutic escape.

Being in the presence of a controlling figure (the top) makes some people feel the kind of safety and protection they felt as a child. Others like the feeling of surrendering themselves, of disappearing into the unavoidable nothingness that comes from relinquishing all power. Still others like earning the approval of a dominant figure or turning their partner into somebody more commanding and powerful.

Command and Control.
Taking the dominant position, on the other hand, provides the thrill that comes from placing yourself above someone else (literally as well as figuratively). You can enjoy the

authority of telling someone what to do, watching them obey, and experiencing the high of "owning" them for a short while. Because when the entirety of your penis is in their body, trust me, you own their attention.

Top/bottom power playing is an exploration of your sexuality and personal boundaries. It's a way to play up excitement and intensity of the sexual experience. It transports you out of judgmental thoughts into territory that widens and deepens your understanding of who you are. It's hard to dredge up judgments about you're every day life when you're in the middle of a passionate, personal sexual odyssey. Playing with power through topping and bottoming is the ultimate form of participation—the key to broadening your experiences.

How To Discover Your Inner Top.

If you've never topped before or tried unsuccessfully because of the emotional blocks we've talked about, it's easy to think that you're not top material. But that isn't true. My bet is that you simply couldn't find your inner top.

So how do you do that? How do you find and cultivate the top within? The best way of doing that is to understand what kind of power you're attracted to and build on what you already like. Power is everywhere during sex and like water to a fish you may not even be aware that it's there, but it is. Let's revisit the simple act of kissing. How could there possibly be a power differential in something so innocent? Let's explore.

How do you find your inner top? By taking your erotic temperature and understanding what kind of sexual power turns you on.

Are you the one who initiated the kiss or the one receiving it? Because the one giving it is exerting power. The one receiving the kiss is submitting to it. Let's say you're on top of him when you kiss him. What do you feel? How does he react? Do you like it? Not so much the kissing part but the part where you're on top. What aspect do you like? Why? Do you want to go further or dial it back? What would make it more arousing? What do you want him to say? What do you want him to do? This is your opportunity to shop the sample sale of your innermost desires. Of course, it can be a little challenging to understand what it is exactly about taking the 'active' role that appeals to you (whether it's kissing or intercourse). That's why you should...

Take Your Erotic Temperature.

In order to understand what it is you like about exerting or submitting to power I want you circle the appropriate temperature for each power play suggestion below. Don't worry about overlapping or contradictory preferences or trying to "identify yourself" either as mostly submissive or mostly dominant. You can, for example, prefer to be submissive during a kiss and dominant during intercourse. Submission

and domination can be traded and played with like cards.
We're looking for opportunities, not labels.

Dominant Power Preferences

I prefer to give than receive.

Cold   Cool   Lukewarm   Warm   HOT

I tend to initiate sex.

Cold   Cool   Lukewarm   Warm   HOT

I like being "on top" during romantic activity like kissing.

Cold   Cool   Lukewarm   Warm   HOT

I like telling my partner what to do in bed.

Cold   Cool   Lukewarm   Warm   HOT

I like exerting control.

Cold   Cool   Lukewarm   Warm   HOT

I like feeling like my partner's protector.

Cold   Cool   Lukewarm   Warm   HOT

I like taking the lead and showing a bit of aggression.

Cold   Cool   Lukewarm   Warm   HOT

I like being powerful and commanding in bed.

Cold   Cool   Lukewarm   Warm   HOT

I like seeing my partner obey my sexual instructions.

Cold   Cool   Lukewarm   Warm   HOT

I like sex a bit on the rough side.

Cold   Cool   Lukewarm   Warm   HOT

I like coming close to verbally insulting my partner in bed.

Cold   Cool   Lukewarm   Warm   HOT

I like the feeling of possessing my partner.

Cold   Cool   Lukewarm   Warm   HOT

I like to partially or fully immobilize my partner with my hands and feet.

Cold   Cool   Lukewarm   Warm   HOT

I like to pinch, squeeze, hold, or otherwise touch my partner in a forceful way.

Cold   Cool   Lukewarm   Warm   HOT

I like doling out "angry" sex.

Cold   Cool   Lukewarm   Warm   HOT

I like to come close to hurting my partner during sex.

Cold   Cool   Lukewarm   Warm   HOT

I like to "punish" my partner with sex.

Cold   Cool   Lukewarm   Warm   HOT

And just to make sure we don't get lop-sided, let's take your erotic temperature on submissiveness…

Submissive Power Preferences

I prefer to receive rather than give.

Cold   Cool   Lukewarm   Warm   HOT

I tend to respond to rather than initiate sex

Cold   Cool   Lukewarm   Warm   HOT

I like being in the bottom during romantic activity like kissing or intercourse.

Cold   Cool   Lukewarm   Warm   HOT

I like being told what to do in bed.

Cold   Cool   Lukewarm   Warm   HOT

I like surrendering control.

Cold   Cool   Lukewarm   Warm   HOT

I like feeling protected by my partner.

Cold   Cool   Lukewarm   Warm   HOT

I like it when my partner takes the lead and shows a bit of aggression.

Cold   Cool   Lukewarm   Warm   HOT

I like it when my partner is powerful and commanding in bed.

Cold   Cool   Lukewarm   Warm   HOT

I like obeying my partner's sexual instructions.

Cold   Cool   Lukewarm   Warm   HOT

I like intercourse a little bit on the rough side.

Cold   Cool   Lukewarm   Warm   HOT

I like it when my partner comes close to verbally insulting me in bed.

Cold   Cool   Lukewarm   Warm   HOT

I like feeling possessed by my partner.

Cold   Cool   Lukewarm   Warm   HOT

I like it when my partner partially or fully immobilizes me with his hands and feet.

Cold   Cool   Lukewarm   Warm   HOT

I like it when my partner pinches, squeezes, holds, or otherwise touches me in a forceful way.

Cold   Cool   Lukewarm   Warm   HOT

I like to be the recipient of "angry" sex.

Cold   Cool   Lukewarm   Warm   HOT

I like it when my partner comes close to hurting me during sex.

Cold   Cool   Lukewarm   Warm   HOT

I like it when my partner acts as if he's punishing me with sex.

Cold   Cool   Lukewarm   Warm   HOT

Free Your Mind, Your Crotch Will Follow.

The point of taking my erotic temperature quiz isn't to label yourself a top or a bottom. It's to understand what aspect of each power differential you're attracted to. Most guys are not one way or the other—a dom top or a helpless bottom. They fall in a spectrum surprisingly influenced by circumstance. Even the Dom-est top is going to think about giving it up for a Chris Hemsworth. And even the most submissive bottom meets guys he could picture himself topping.

The spectrum of power preference is influenced by mood and environment. You will find yourself, as most guys do, sometimes acting like a teenage girl or a macho prick, depending on the circumstance. Masculinity, femininity, dominance and submissiveness are rarely mutually exclusive. Be in touch with both as both will serve you well.

Now, take a few days to really sort through the choices you made on this quiz and come to an understanding of what you like. Sometimes the shyest guys have a secret wish to dominate and sometimes the most dominating personalities yearn to be taught a few lessons.

The point of this exercise is to get a clear picture of what turns you on so you can start crafting a better vision of how you want to top. Let this be the start of a conversation that allows you to have fun, push boundaries, and explore some areas of your own psychology. But mostly, let it be about forming what type of 'topulinity' works for you. Don't get stuck on the "right" answer—there is none. The only "right" answer is the one you feel comfortable with.

When I say take a few days to sort through the choices you made, what I mean is to reflect on them and take them to their natural conclusion. For example, if you circled "Luke-warm" (or warmer than that) on "I like to tell my partner what to do in bed" ask yourself a few questions: Why? What about that turns me on? How do I feel when I make a request? How do I feel when he complies? What about this scenario arouses me?

Do this self-exploration on every statement you circled "lukewarm" or hotter. Get to know yourself better. A better understanding will help shape your topulinity. Again, the point isn't to take on somebody else's definition of how power should be expressed, but to discover different expressions that work for you.

Exploring a new dimension in your sex life means playing with that thing between your ears, not your legs. So as you experiment with different activities, embrace the power-playing role you take on and understand what drives it.

The Different Types Of Topping That Receivers Prefer.

One way of getting comfortable with the kind of top you want to be is to understand what guys who bottom tend to like. And that is completely dependent on the receiver's personality. What one guy thinks is a hit another guy would give it a miss. Fundamentally, the choice is between rough-ness and tenderness. Let's take a look:

The Command & Control Top Who Gives A Back Alley Pounding.

This is the guy you see almost exclusively in porn. He's locked, cocked and ready to rock. Your wishes as the bottom mean nothing to him. You are there to be his receptacle. Does it hurt? Shut up it's supposed to hurt. WHACK!

There is something to be said about the junkyard dog's energy compared to the teacup poodle but that doesn't mean everyone wants to be on the receiving end of that. But many do, as you're about to read in these quotes I gathered from a variety of gay forums:

"I want them dumber than dirt and fucking like a runaway jack-hammer."

• • •

"I want a top who's verbal, aggressive, and knows how to be dirty. A guy who knows what positions he likes and can flip you from one to the other in a second.

• • •

"I like my tops to be muscular, taller than me and very strong because they usually control the pace so they should have the right stamina to do so. I quite like being submissive."

• • •

"I like a guy to start slow and passionate then pick up and go wolverine on me."

• • •

"A good top is one who can take control mentally and physically. This means being big enough and strong enough to push, pull, and drag me around. Strong enough to hold me where he wants me and make sure I'm not going to be able to get away too easily. Also somebody who mentally takes over. Not a pussy who's afraid to hurt me. Yes, go gentle at first to make sure I'm comfortable and not in pain, but after we're relaxed a bit more, let the beast loose!"

• • •

"I love being shown who is boss."

•••

What turns me on the most is when a man knows what he wants and takes it without any question. I like it rough mostly. I like my ass slapped and a man moaning pushes me overboard. I like it verbal. I'm very sexual and prefer a man that can LAST as well. That's what I need. A man that knows my limits and yet at times knows that sometimes no really does mean yes."

The Tender Top

I once overheard a straight couple arguing about their sex life. The guy says, "Do you know what the difference is between fucking and making love?" No, said the wife, enlighten me. "Making love is what the woman's doing as the guy fucks her."

My point, and I do have one, is that if the dom top is about fucking, then the tender top is about making love. Unlike the porn stereotype, this is the guy who really does care about his bottom partner and treats him with respect and kindness. Here's a sampling from various forums extolling the virtues of the tender top:

"I want a top to dominate me but also one who doesn't treat me like a bitch. While yes, I prefer the passive role as I like a dominant guy who DOES take control, I'm not a bitch."

•••

"I hate a guy who just pounds. Look if I wanted to fuck a jackhammer or a hamster on crack, I would. But that's just me. Everyone likes it differently. What one person says is a great top is another guy's nightmare of a top. When I am topping I like to get a clue what my bottom likes based on the sounds he's making during foreplay and sex. For me it's a full body experience."

•••

"As a top, I've been told (more often than not), that someone had the hottest sex of their lives with me. Not bragging here (well maybe a bit). It's really simple, I think…you give the bottom exactly what they need, want and crave. You fulfill the fantasy…you find out and pay attention to what turns them on and then you deliver—whether it's a hard, pounding, sweaty fucking or a slow and passionate lovemaking; whether it's dominant and aggressive or sensuous and mutual)."

•••

"I try and make the bottom enjoy it more than I do, and I enjoy fucking A LOT, so my job is to make the bottom have a better time than I am. Sure, I love fucking and trust me, I will do ANYTHING to get my dick up your ass, but I also treat my bottoms with respect and care."

•••

"I would have to say that my success at being a good top is figuring out what my partner likes and then incorporating that into what comes naturally for me to make us both happy. To me it's definitely a team effort."

...

"My ideal top isn't just physical. It's about emotional, and passionate love making. Give and take, making love furiously, intensely. No matter how you cut it, a man opening himself up for another man to enter him is the ultimate in submission. I want my man to dominate me, but I am not a passive bottom. When I have a man inside me, I feel that I have the essence of that man inside me. And even though he is the aggressor, he also needs my body to achieve the ultimate release. It has to be making love, not just mindless fucking, or rape...at least for me. You have to care for your partner, even if he is a total stranger. You are sharing that moment in your life with that man in the most intimate way physically. You may say lighten up but for me to allow another man to enter me, I do not take it so lightly. I want to enjoy myself to the fullest (and be completely full with him)."

The Romanticized Version of A Dom Top

This is the idealized mix between a good power driller and the dreamy husband who knows how to make love. Get a load of these high-wire descriptions:

What makes a good top? Stamina and ferocity. Selfless

devotion to the thrill for the bottom, and outrageous pride in proving himself the most agile and powerful man imaginable. A generous conqueror. The ability to be vocal helps - not so much verbal, but for god's sake howl a little man! A truly accomplished top is athletic and agile and certain of himself. A brutal force that moves things around with grace that equals a tiger playing with his prey before going in for the kill.

A good top pulls you up, face to face, and kisses you with the same brutal passion, sucking the wind out of you while drilling as deep as possible. A truly good top pushes everything down through his cock as an extension of his mind, and he has his partner's ass begging, pulling, and kneading at his cock, and then responds to that with purpose and a warrior's devotion to spilling every last drop of his testosterone in, on and all the fuck over you, and not stop until he's brought you to the edge so many times that you literally explode for him. And then he has to know how to finish the job, licking, tasting, kissing, and pull you close and let you feel the EXACT same power, near lethal, as you stroke and hold and are tender. Fearless strength of purpose, protective, possessive and just waiting long enough for you to catch your breath before he gets that look that threatens and thrills - ready to start all over.

...

A good top for me fucks with his entire body not just his cock ... I hate the word dominance ... I want to be enveloped and surrounded by his body ... even when I'm at my most sluttiest

I want a lot of foreplay and touching …I don't have the most amazing body so I like a top who gets off on my worshipping his … maybe I don't hate the word dominate so much … because a good top for me will instinctively know how even when just sitting next to him… putting one of his legs on top of mine makes me feel wanted and warm … I like a top who knows that even in the middle of a hardcore pounding it feels good to have him lean down and hold me so I can feel his chest muscles against my back … he knows that just because I came… doesn't mean he has to stop…

What Kind Of Top Do You Want To Be?

This is an important question you need to answer for yourself. A dom top? A tender top? Something in between? Here's how to choose: Don't. Let it choose you. What characteristics of a grab-it-and-growl dom top do you like? Some? None? All? Express it in your lovemaking. What characteristics of a tender top resonate with you? All, none or some? Again, absorb what feels right so you can express it authentically.

And now that we've got your topulinity straightened out let's tackle the #1 reason that stops guys from topping. Hey, wait. Does my finger smell funny?

CHAPTER TWO

What's That Smell?
The Dirty Reason That Stops You From Topping

Some Real-World Tactics For Overcoming Hygiene Worries

The biggest obstacle that prevents men from inserting their prized possession on those they find attractive is the fear that they're going to have a Third Encounter With The Brown Kind. Seeing and smelling your own shit can leave you a little nauseous so it stands to reason than seeing or smelling someone else's is going to be even worse. Walking into an unclean public restroom is enough to give even raging tops a moment of pause about where they're putting their penises.

This can be further exacerbated if you're a clean freak or have bouts with germ phobia. Let's be clear and not dance around the subject: You are sticking your penis into a cavity whose primary function is to eliminate feces from the body. This is not a comforting thought for most of us. So how do experienced tops get over it? What do they do? How do they think? Is there a recognized strategy for overcoming the fear and revulsion that topping might expose you to undesirable sights and smells?

Yes. Let's take them one by one. They're actually related to each other. Like ropes hanging in the jungle, you can mentally swing from one to the other to get to your destination faster.

Put It In Perspective. His Anus Ain't Heinous.

Nobody but a drunk newbie is going to bottom without being reasonably clean down there, so the chances that you're going to encounter some kind of shit bomb is highly unlikely if next to impossible (mostly because the anal canal doesn't store feces). That leaves the reality of an occasionally unpleasant whiff and the possibility of a small stain. Now you can FREAK OUT or you can react calmly by thinking something like, "Yup, I recognize that smell. It'll go away pretty quickly" and keep about your business.

Keep Your Eye On The Doughnut And Not On The Hole.

Where do you want to put your attention—on the possibility of experiencing uncleanliness or the certainty of volcanic pleasure? Where you decide to put your psychic energy has consequences. You can concentrate on the anticipation of an off-putting smell or sight or you can concentrate on how good something is going to feel. One is going to kill your boner; the other is going to strengthen it. Concentrate your attention on his anus as a penis pleasurer, the route to fantastic sensations and psychological thrills. These rewards make the negatives of a whiff or a sight pale in comparison. It's like comparing a small and temporary 'yuck' reaction to a huge and long-lasting pleasure.

Practice Denial. It Ain't Just A River In Egypt.

There is great power in pretending something you don't want isn't there. A great deal of guys simply block out any images or thoughts of the anus as a method of elimination and concentrate only on its erotic appeal. There is much to commend this strategy because it short-circuits aversion. Denial is made easier by your partner bottom taking pre-cautions—through bathing, showering, doing a little finger-mopping or full-on douching. Denial is also aided and abetted by the urgency of wanting to fuck. A hard dick has no conscience and it will certainly make you lose your sense of sight and smell if it has to.

Accept The Trade-off.

Everything is a trade-off including sex. Especially sex. A lot of guys simply accept the occasional smell or stain as the cost of doing business. There is a lot of risk attached to sex—gonorrhea, syphilis, HPV, herpes and of course HIV. When you stop and think about it, these risks make the possibility of experiencing a lapse of hygiene positively quaint. Of all the things to worry about during sex, this should rank somewhere around page 3.

Ask Your Partner If He's Clean Before The Pants Come Off.

The best way to deal with a bad situation is to prevent it from happening in the first place. Asking your partner a simple question can minimize negative experiences. Don't be shy. All you have to say is, "Are you clean enough down there for us to play?" An ounce of prevention is worth a pound of "eeews."

As you can see, men who top use various coping strategies to deal with the hygiene problem. Different situations will call for different coping strategies but it's a safe bet that combining these methods will get you, ahem, over the hump.

Another way of dealing with it is to simply become more informed about how the body works. The more you understand about the anus the less scary it becomes. While at first it can be a little unsettling to read about how, say, the anal canal works, you will find yourself grossing out less and less to the point where it simply doesn't bother you much at all.

In that spirit, I am now going to give you a primer on how butts work. The fear of leaving muddy tire tracks on the sheets or your partner's penis is based on a misconception that feces are stored in the rectum. In fact, they are not. Feces are stored in the sigmoid colon, which sits above the rectum. The only time your rectum fills with stool is when the sigmoid colon fills up and needs to release it.

Through a combination of anatomical structure, neural switches and reflex triggers it is impossible for stool to remain in your rectum. Now, often there is residue, for sure, and we'll talk about that later in the book. For now, know that your rectum, the place that will lovingly hold and pet your penis, is a pipeline, not a storage device. It is the Panama Canal between the sigmoid colon and your sphincter. Ships can only pass through; they cannot anchor.

Let's take a look at why. It'll be helpful to see a diagram of how the sigmoid colon (where the last stages of fecal matter are produced) attaches to the rectum. Click here for some enlightening diagrams: http://bit.ly/1Pjc4IP.

The sigmoid colon releases waste (stool) to the rectum when the body is ready for elimination and only when it is ready. There are several ways the body makes sure that things don't 'slip' into the rectum accidentally. First, the juncture between the sigmoid colon and the rectum lies at ninety degrees. The sigmoid colon is horizontal where it meets the rectum, which lies on a more vertical plane. This sharp angle stops feces from entering the rectum on their own. "Security" is reinforced by a sphincter muscle between the sigmoid and the rectum (Christ, how many sphincters do we have in our bodies!). In its natural state this sphincter is constricted and thus acts as the gatekeeper. It remains tightly shut unless it receives a command from headquarters.

As fecal content grows in the sigmoid colon it exerts pressure on this sphincter muscle. This triggers one of many involuntary "defecation reflexes" and signals the sigmoid sphincter to open up and let the fecal content into the rectum. The entry of feces into the rectum distends the rectal wall. There, stretch receptors trigger signals to the descending and sigmoid colon to increase peristalsis (the involuntary constriction and relaxation of the muscles, creating wavelike movements that push the fecal contents forward). These "waves" of movement pass through all the way to the anus, causing the puborectal sling to loosen, straightening the S curve in your rectum, and causing the internal sphincter (remember him, the one who doesn't obey your orders to relax?) to completely relax (the bastard!).

But defecation only happens once you release the external sphincter, which you have conscious control of. When you can't find a bathroom (and you'd rather not relieve yourself on the carpet) you can clench your external sphincter to keep it from happening. You will also be aided by the sling, which acts as "continence muscle" that stops you from farting or taking a shit in the middle of a cocktail party. When you need to go but can't, the sling responds to the pressure by contracting, which holds the feces back until you have the opportunity to find a bathroom.

Nice, huh?

Interesting Aside.

If you're able to prevent defecation long enough by consciously clenching your external sphincter, the stool in the rectum is often returned to the colon by reverse peristalsis, temporarily reducing pressure in the rectum (deactivating the stretch receptors). The stool is then stored in the sigmoid colon until the transverse and descending colon, which connects to the sigmoid from above, triggers the next peristalsis movement. You only want to delay defecation in cases when there are no bathrooms or you're stuck in some circumstance that prevents you from accessing one (accepting an Oscar for Best Supporting Bottom, for example). If defecation is delayed long enough, the fecal matter may harden and oh, dear, you'll get as constipated as Ru Paul out of drag.

So what does all this have to do with topping? A lot. First, understanding the process of elimination helps reassure you that the rectum does not store feces. This should put you at ease: Your partner will not release a shit bomb if you top him.

Second, there are parallels between elimination and insertion (something you need to know about if you're going to top well). If you want objects to make a smooth entrance, it behooves you to understand how they make a graceful exit. For example, let's take that sling inside you. It pulls the lower rectum forward toward the belly button up to 90 degrees, creating an S curve. The tighter the sling, the more pronounced the S curve. The sling prevents things from leaving the rectum (it's one of the reasons you strain in the toilet) and prevents things from entering it (it blocks the penis by greeting it with the rectal wall). So let's study how the sling releases for elimination because your partner can use that knowledge to release it during insertion.

During defecation the sling loosens so much it decreases the S curve from almost ninety degrees to 15 degrees (almost straight) causing the external sphincter to relax involuntarily. Those power bottoms that can take cargo so easily? They've mastered the loosening of the sling during sex, so bottoming becomes a pain free breeze. While you cannot consciously relax the puborectal sling, there are positions that naturally straighten it. Positions like the ones you take when you go to the bathroom.

Normally, you sit on the toilet with hips and knees at about a right angle. It's known as the "Catcher's position" because it's so close to the position baseball catchers take during a game. But since toilets were only invented in the nineteenth century, a good part of the world doesn't use the "catcher's position" for elimination. They use a "squatting toilet" (fancy for a hole in the ground). This forces you to squat all the way down to your ankles.

Many proctologists believe that the catcher's position we use in the western world creates bowel movement problems because it does not sufficiently loosen the puborectal sling. This keeps the S curve fairly pronounced, causing many people to strain in the bathroom. In fact research shows people strain three times greater in a sitting position than a squatting one.

Whoa, whoa! Enough of this shit! What does all this discussion about defecation postures have to do with topping? Again, the S curve that makes it harder for things to go out your butt is the same S curve that makes things hard for things to go in it. The "catcher's position" you take on the toilet is most like the missionary position in bed—on your back with knees raised at ninety degrees to your torso. That straightens the S sling a bit but not by a lot. But the squatting position significantly straightens out the S curve. And that is why you should start topping by having your partner squat on top of you rather than taking the missionary position. You will be shocked at how much easier your penis goes in this way. Why? Because squatting releases the sling, which straightens the S curve.

This also brings us to another point worth mentioning. Many guys feel like they have to defecate when a penis enters their rectum. Why is that? If you review the early part of this chapter you'll remember that the rectum has "stretch sensors." When the rectum is full, stretch receptors fire, giving you the feeling that you have to take a dump. When a penis enters the rectum, it sets off these stretch sensors, in the way your cat might set off the fire alarm. In other words, that feeling that you have to take a dump? It's a false alarm. This sensation will wane as your rectum learns to re-interpret the presence of a penis. It is not possible for you to have a bowel movement during sex, even if it feels like you need to.

The Best Way To Get Your Partner Clean.

This section of the book is really written for your partner. If you have a boyfriend/husband/regular sex partner hand it to him. He'll get cleaner than a floor licked by a cat. But it's also for you, too, if you're versatile or want to be clean enough to bottom.

Okay, let's get started. Although the anal canal and rectum are not storage devices for feces, it's not exactly like you can eat off your anus like it were Aunt Edna's kitchen floor. If you stick a finger up your bum (go ahead, I'll wait), it's mostly clean when you pull it out but it won't win the starring role in a Purell commercial. Like a good courtroom lawyer, you will always find evidence that a grime was committed. And if you do some finger excavating to root out the brown evil you will note that while there are no sizable fudge brownies, there might be sludge and even the occasional booger. How can you get yourself clean? Like most problems, the best way to solve this one is to avoid it in the first place.

Improve Your Diet.

Does your underwear look like Jackson Pollock aimed his ass at the canvas and yelled, "FIRE!"? Does your rectum look like it hosted a NASCAR event? If you do a little finger mopping up there and come out with more than just a faint residue (there will always be a little) you can bet the culprit is your diet. Specifically, you are not eating enough fiber or drinking enough water. Fiber is responsible for:

• **Keeping your shit together.**

Soluble fiber (like bananas) dissolves in water but isn't digested, so it absorbs excess liquid in the colon, forms a thick gel and adds lots of bulk to your feces as it parades up Intestinal Hill and down to Rectum Road. Like most gay pride parades, it picks up hitch-hiking stragglers. It also softens and pushes through impacted fecal matter. The fiber, I mean, not gay pride. Though you could make a case for that, too.

• **Shaping your shit.**

Ever see those old videos of Tokyo transit police pushing passengers in with those sort of giant Schwab sticks so they can squeeze more people into the train? That's what insoluble fiber (like broccoli) does. Since it won't dissolve in water and can't be absorbed by the body, it passes through your stomach essentially intact, compacting brown "passengers" into the intestinal train and giving them the best shape to go through the colon and out your anus without breaking off and leaving unwanted specimens.

Fiber Is Your Ticket To Cleanliness.

By "bulking up" waste matter and shaping it for easier transit, fiber ensures that feces leave the rectum and anal canal virtually intact, leaving you with just a smidge of sludge, a slight residue that's easy to clean with just a little finger mopping. The problem is that you most likely suffer from a serious fiber deficiency. How do I know? Because the American Dietetic Association says so. Take a look at their stats:

Recommended Fiber Intake For Men: 30-38 grams*
Average Fiber Intake For Men: 10-15 grams

* Some experts believe it should be as high as 60 grams.

Think about this—the average guy eats less than half the recommended amount of fiber! And then they wonder why their rectum looks like a landfill? There is no clean rectum without fiber adding bulk to the waste in your colorectal system and shaping it for easy transit out of your anus. Your mission, should you decide to accept a clean rectum, is to consistently eat about 40 grams of fiber a day. Here are a few tips on how to do that through diet alone:

1. Eat Foods That Are High In Soluble Fiber.

Soluble fiber dissolves easily in water, forming a gel-like substance that absorbs water and makes the bowel contents stickier, which binds more waste to it. This slows the speed that foods move through the stomach, making you feel fuller longer and helping you maintain or lose weight. The slow transit time is incredibly helpful if you suffer from diarrhea. Soluble fiber also softens your stool so it can pass through your system more comfortably. It also lowers the levels of LDL cholesterol and improves your ability to control your body's blood glucose level. What's not to like? Examples of soluble fiber: bananas, apples, brown rice, white beans.

2. Eat Foods That Are High In Insoluble Fiber.

Insoluble fiber doesn't dissolve in water. In fact, it passes through your intestines intact and that's why it increases stool bulk. It's also why it accelerates transit time, relieving constipation. Examples of insoluble fiber: Kale, lentils, pears.

Now, if you're reading this carefully you'll note the following:

- Soluble fiber slows transit time, relieving diarrhea.

- Insoluble fiber speeds transit time, relieving constipation.

How can this be? Will fiber confuse your body, making your rectum shit or go blind? No, soluble and insoluble fiber are the answer to both diarrhea and constipation because they regulate digestion for smooth bowel movements, which is critical to keeping you clean for bottoming.

Most fiber-rich foods contain both soluble and insoluble fiber, yet most food labels—and health sites—don't make a distinction between the two and simply list the overall fiber content of a food. How can you find out which foods have the highest soluble and/or insoluble fiber? By clicking on this terrific chart by commonsensehealth.com. It's by far the most useful fiber chart I've ever seen. Use it to balance the two types of fiber in your diet. You can also calculate the fiber in your meals by using WebMD's dietary fiber calculator. Click here: http://www.webmd.com/diet/healthtool-fiber-meter.

Porn Star Bottoms All Say That What They Eat Affects Their Ability To Bottom.

There is remarkable agreement among those in the porn industry that what you eat—and when—has a dramatic effect on the clean factor. Here's what a famous (or rather infamous) porn star bottom told us:

"1 to 2 days prior to the shoot date, you want to eat as light as possible. Breakfast for me would have been an egg hard-boiled, and lunch grilled chicken, and a side salad, and I would probably do the same thing for dinner. So the majority

of that diet is lean meats and fibers, no carbohydrates. I drink water and teas, and stay away from carbonated sodas because they would also – the last thing you want to do before a scene is eat or drink anything that would make you gassy."

What If Diet Alone Can't Get You To Your Fiber Goals?

It's much better to get fiber through your diet, but this being Fast Food Nation, it won't hurt for you to take fiber supplements. The main drawback to supplements is that they lack the vitamins, minerals, and antioxidants you get from eating high fiber foods like fruits, whole grains, and beans.

The kind of fiber supplement (psyllium, methylcellulose, wheat dextrin) or brand (Konsyl, Metamucil, Citrucel, etc.) you take or the forms you take it (pills, powder, caplets, gummy bears) don't really matter. They all behave in pretty much the same way. The most common source for fiber supplements is psyllium, which comes from the seeds of a plant species called Plantago Ovata. When the husk of these seeds is placed in water they expand in size and take on a gel-like consistency. This gel-like mass soaks up water and adds bulk to your stool.

In powder form these supplements taste like sawdust sprinkled with sweeteners. Fortunately, many come in pills and capsules, which is good because I know how much you like to swallow. I kid. Start with the minimum dosage in the bottle and work yourself up. S-L-O-W-L-Y. Too much fiber at one time can make you bloat, pass gas and create unenviable digestive issues. Remember, bedrooms are No Fart Zones. You don't want your partners dying of auto-not-so-erotic asphyxiation. A couple of things you should know about taking fiber supplements:

- Spread your fiber intake throughout the day. Don't take the full dose only at night. Spread it evenly throughout the morning, afternoon and bedtime.

- Take medications at least one hour before fiber supplements or two hours after. Fiber is known to absorb certain medicines, diverting them from your body.

- Drink lots of water. Did I say a lot? Because I meant A LOT. Taking fiber without water is like bottoming without lube. It's going to hurt like hell. Drink at least eight ounces of water with every dosage.

What If You Have Stomach Problems?
A lot of gay men have IBS (Irritable Bowel Syndrome) that make their rectums a little more, ahm, messier than they like. If this seems embarrassingly true for you, I'd recommend three things:

1. The Fiber Supplement Proven To Help IBS.
Calcium polycarbophil has been proven to regulate diarrhea, constipation, bloating and abdominal pain in patients suffering with IBS. Choose from the fol-

lowing brands and work up slowly from one gram a day to six: Fibercon, Konsyl, Fiber-tab, Fiber-Lax or Equalactin.

Even if you don't have IBS you might consider using calcium polycarbophil, a synthetic form of fiber rather than psyllium, which is naturally occurring. You'd think the natural stuff would be better for you but calcium polycarbophil runs less of a risk of interacting with gut bacteria and producing unwanted gas. I guess it's the drag queen equivalent of fiber supplements—more real in its fakeness than even the genuine stuff.

2. A Prebiotic.

A prebiotic is essentially food for probiotics (the "good bacteria" in your gut), which promote digestive health. The one that has the most science behind it is Inulin. Because it's not digested or absorbed in the stomach it settles in the bowels where the "good" bacteria (probiotics) feed on it, thus improving bowel function (inulin is a natural compound found in a wide variety of fruits, vegetables and herbs). Brands with inulin include Metamucil Clear & Natural, Fiber-Choice, and Benefiber. Take as directed. Inulin stays in your gut and helps the "good" intestinal bacteria grow. You might want to consider taking psyllium along with inulin. Some studies show great promise in using both substances to help treat IBS.

3. A Probiotic.

Probiotics are "good" bacteria that reduce the growth of harmful bacteria and promote a healthy digestive system. Is that vague enough for you? While it's true that probiotics are recognized as beneficial to the digestive system, there are 400 types of probiotic bacteria in your gut. The best known of the pro-biotics is Lactobacillus acidophilus, which is found in yogurt with live cultures. It is not known which probiotics (alone or in combination) work to actually remedy a malady like bloating or diarrhea. There is only one probiotic that shows great promise for people with IBS or moderate-to-severe stomach problems. It's called Bifidobacterium infantis 35624. Several well-respected studies like this one (http://www.ncbi.nlm.nih.gov/pubmed/15765388) from the National Center Of Biotechnology Information show that it significantly reduces abdominal pain/discomfort, bloating/distention, and bowel movement difficulty.

There is only one brand that sells Bifidobacterium infantis 35624. It's called Align, and it's sold pretty much at drug stores everywhere. Unfortunately, it's the costliest probiotic out there.

You Can Tell How Dirty Your Rectum Is Without Inserting A Finger.

Look down. Not at your underwear; the toilet. The size,

shape and color of your poo will determine how much residue is left in your rectum. Let's start with the sound your stools make as they hit the toilet water. I'd like to quote Dr. Mehmet Oz's unforgettable observation:

"You want to hear what the stool, the poop, sounds like when it hits the water. If it sounds like a bombardier, you know, 'plop, plop, plop,' that's not right because it means you're constipated. It means the food is too hard by the time it comes out. It should hit the water like a diver from Acapulco hits the water [swoosh]."

After hearing the swoosh sound (hopefully) look down. Your stool should be an S shape. That signifies that the stool is firm enough that it doesn't break off in little pieces, but soft enough so it doesn't hurt coming out.

Don't worry about the frequency of your bowel movement. It can be as often as three times a day or as infrequent as three times per week. There is no normal; only what's normal for you. You're better off paying attention to what the bowel movement smells like than anything else. Healthy bowel movements should not force the next person using the bathroom to wear a biohazard suit. Strong- or foul-smelling stool means there's something wrong with what you're eating.

The Fibrous Conclusion.
Eating enough fiber is the only way to make sure that you

can bottom without stains or odors. Fiber improves the passage of feces through your colon so that it comes out soft but firm, sweeping up stragglers and leaving no remnants in the rectum as it exits your anus. Fiber is not going to make the boys at Brita raise a glass of your butt spit and say, "Now THAT'S filtered water!" But it will ensure that you'll never have an ugly "shit bomb" episode that scars you —and your lacy white curtains—for life.

CHAPTER THREE

This Won't Hurt A Bit. How To Get Your Partner To Relax His Sphincter.

A Most Ingenious Method For Pain-Free Penetration

Pain, or the fear of pain, is probably the biggest reason your potential partners shy away from bottoming. Consequently, "pain management" is going to be your biggest challenge as a top, especially if you're bigger than average. You're going to have to learn how to help your partner relax or the only thing you're going to top is a pot.

In this chapter I'm going to show you specific techniques that will allow your partner to experience the ecstasy of bottoming without any of the pain he's come to fear or associate with it. Let's start by getting into the right mental space.

How "Anticipatory Pain" Can Make Your Butt Tighter Than Two Coats Of Paint.

"Anticipatory pain" is a psychological term for the expectation of pain. It speaks to the emotional and physical consequences of this expectation. For example, if your partner is convinced that bottoming for you will be painful, his body will tense up in the expectation of it. The more he believes that bottoming will hurt, the tenser his body will get. His butt will clench for its safety as hard as it can. This expectation of pain contributes greatly to an inability to relax. If he's convinced that bottoming for you is going to hurt like hell, how in God's pajamas is he going to be relaxed enough to enjoy it? Imagine telling someone, "This is going to hurt worse than a motor-powered root canal, so just relax." Right. That's helpful.

> With the right conditioning anal muscles can relax enough to easily accommodate a large penis without any pain whatsoever..

But wait, your partner says! He's heard horror stories from friends and hell, it hurts even when you stick your pinky up there—how could a penis NOT hurt going in? Here's how: Because the entire anus, from the sphincter to the anal canal to the rectum, is made up of incredibly supple, flexible muscle and tissue that, with the right conditioning, can stretch and expand way beyond its current size without causing harm or pain. To get a sense of the flexibility in your puborectal region, know this: During rectal surgery your anus can be safely stretched to the point that the surgeon's hand can easily pass through the anal canal.

Let's just hope the surgeon doesn't get an attack of jazz hands during the procedure.

With the right conditioning anal muscles can relax enough to easily accommodate a penis without any pain whatsoever. You see the evidence of this on your computer's hard drive or your Internet browser—where you store, bookmark and view your favorite porn. If you learn anything from porn (other than you like way too much of it!) it's this: With the right approach, you can painlessly take in guys who are hung like the Florida panhandle.

Okay, so how do you get your partner to relax? Let's start with something that might surprise you.

You Have Two Sphincters.

You may only have one anus but two connecting sphincters surround it. They are distinct but overlapping bands of muscle tissue. And while they serve the exact same function (regulating grand openings and final close-outs) they go about it in different ways. You are most familiar with the external sphincter because you can order it to tighten and release. Here, try it. Squinch your starfish by using the muscles to stop yourself from peeing. Got it? Tighten, release, tighten, release. Now, this time with feeling! Tighten, release. Now do five fast tightens. Get it? You can boss that part of your butt around. Feel like taking a crap but there's no bathroom around? No problem. You can will your external sphincter not to open. At least for a while.

But the internal sphincter? You can't tell it to do shit. And I mean that in every sense of the word. You are not its boss.

Like your blood pressure and heartbeat, you cannot directly control it.

Do this: Put your hands in front of you as if you're praying. Now intertwine your fingers down to the webbing and press your palms together as tight as you can. Now keep everything connected and completely relax both hands. Notice the small opening between the side of your thumb and your index finger? This is the opening to your anus. If somebody tried to poke their finger through that opening it would feel snug but it'd go in pretty easy.

Now tighten both hands as hard as you can. The left hand is the internal sphincter you cannot directly control. The right hand is the external sphincter you can. Keeping the left hand tight as a drum, completely relax your right hand. Your right hand (external sphincter) is relaxed so a *slight* opening was created. But your left hand (internal sphincter) is so tight that it won't let a poking finger through very easily.

Welcome to bottoming's first dilemma: The left hand doesn't know what the right hand is doing. Or more accurately, the left hand doesn't *care* what the right hand is doing. The internal and external sphincter can and often do work independently of each other. In order to make penetration smooth and effortless *both* sphincters have to get on the same page. Okay, so the sphincters are pain point #1. Now, let's talk about...

Pain Point #2: His Puborectal Sling.

As stated before, the puborectal sling is a strong ring of supportive muscle that creates a curve in the rectum. It pulls the lower end of the rectum toward your belly button before it straightens out to eventually become the anal canal, which is the passageway from your sphincter to the rectum.

The more the sling pulls the lower rectum toward the navel, the more pronounced your S curve will be. Why would that create pain? Because unless you find a way to straighten the S curve your penis will ram the rectal wall at up to ninety degrees and make your partner think he's getting stabbed on the inside with a bat.

Let's do an experiment. Raise your left hand, palm down. Now poke the palm with your right index finger. This is the penis hitting the rectal wall caused by the S curve. Now move your palm up to ninety degrees (as if you were shaking somebody's hand) and poke it with your index finger the way you did before. You can't. Your finger glides up your palm. That's what bottoming will feel like if you straighten out your S curve.

Now, there is a third point of pain. It's located across the entire puborectal region, and a simple law of nature causes it.

Pain Point # 3: The Law Of Insertion.

Your body automatically contracts when you insert something into it. That's just a fact. The puborectal region is not used to being penetrated. It will interpret the penetrating object as an invading army that must be repelled. Never mind the sphincter and the sling (sounds like a new Disney fairy tale, doesn't it? *"The Sphincter & The Sling"*). Wait. Where was I? Oh, yes, <u>all</u> the muscles, fibers and tissues in the area will contract when you insert a foreign object and make it exceedingly difficult for your partner to bottom for you. These contractions are simply the body trying to protect itself. We'll talk later about how to neutralize this natural reaction, but for now...

Let's Review.

You have three potential points of pain:

1. The Internal And External Sphincters.

They work together (and apart) to keep things in or out. Sometimes they work independently of each other, which is a bummer because it makes complete relaxation a bit trickier. Think of your hands clasped together tightly. If one hand loosens but the other doesn't, it's harder to get a finger through the hole. If both hands loosen the finger slides in easily. It's fairly easy to relax your external sphincter because it obeys conscious command. The internal sphincter? Not so much. Your partner's challenge, as a bottom, is to relax *both* sphincters so that a penis can get through them without causing pain. Your challenge, as a top, is to help your partner do that.

2. The S Curve Caused By The Puborectal Sling.

Even if you get past the gatekeeping sphincters, you have to deal with the S curve in your rectum caused by the pubo-rectal sling. It forces the lower end of the rectum to curve toward the navel, thus creating a situation where the incoming penis hits the anal wall almost perpendicularly. The pain will make your partner wish impotence on you. Think of a highway guardrail curving into the middle of the road. Less road and more guardrail means the car is bound to hit the barrier and cause some damage.

3. The Puborectal Contractions.

The body knows that the best way to repel an invading force is to shut everything down tightly. Because the puborectal region is only used to things going out of it, the attempt to put something into it is going to be met with withering skepticism. Muscles in the surrounding area will clamp down hard and make you pay dearly for your impertinence.

These are the three pain points that will make your bottom partner stop the proceedings unless he, or you, addresses them. Fortunately, we are about to do that.

How To Get Your Partner To Relax His Sphincter.

Obviously, you can't do it for him, but you can do several things that will make it a lot easier for him to relax his sphincter muscles. Let's start by helping him concentrate on desire, rather than fear, of your hard dick.

Remember we talked about "anticipatory pain" and the body's natural "clamp down" reaction to having something inserted into it? Well, you're going to set off both the mental and physical triggers if you try to get inside him too quickly or too forcefully. If you come at him like you're about to stage a rape his sphincter will tighten so much it'll be able to skin a fart.

From an emotional stand-point you have to heat up his desire so much that his body aches for your hard dick to be inside him. *Aches.* Once you engage his emotions his body will follow through. If he wants you in the worse way, his legs will begin to part and his sphincter will start to quiver with the right kind of anticipation—pleasure, not pain.

Getting him to that level of desire is actually pretty easy if you know how to work it. Working it doesn't mean slamming it into him. It means teasing him with your hard-on. It means letting him feel the heat of your hardness between his legs and *on but not in* his anus. It means getting on top and kissing him passionately so that he can feel the excitement of being underneath your body. The best way of bringing out somebody's submissiveness is to let him experience the power of your body.

That power is best seen and experienced from below, looking up, so as you heat up the play make sure you're on top of him a good deal of the time. Your partner loves male bodies (hello! He's about to bottom for you!) so play that up. He also loves male energy so this isn't the time to girl out and tell him how fabulous he would look on your chenille pillow if only he had the right haircut.

Your goal is to tease him, not scare him. That means being strong in the way you lift him, but not rough so he thinks you're going to hurt him. It means showing strength, not force. Inten-

> Be appealingly assertive not aggressively threatening or you're going to turn off guys worried about their safety, masculinity or both.

sity, not coercion. Assertiveness, not aggression. You want to do this for a couple of reasons. First, if you're too rough, too dominant, or too forceful you'll come across as dangerous. While I acknowledge that some guys like that, the vast majority of gay men do not want to feel threatened in bed. You can be in charge in a way that makes you beguiling or in a way that makes you feared.

There's another reason not to cross the boundary from appealingly assertive to aggressively threatening—the closer you are to the line the more you're going to turn off a partner who's having qualms about what bottoming means to his identity as a man. The more you act like he's your bitch, the more you're going to trigger his fear that bottoming will feminize him.

The best way to bring out his desire to have you inside of him is to *simulate* bottoming before proceeding to the real thing. Get on top of him. Gently make him feel your heat, smell your essence, and feel your hardness. Put lube in his hands, place them underneath his ass and gently thrust your penis into them as if it were his anus. He'll feel how smoothly it glides through his hands. He'll feel the strength and the firmness and imagine it going inside him.

Bottoming, like any sex act, is half physical, half psychological. If you want him to truly enjoy bottoming, give him a simulated experience of what it's like to be "taken." A hard penis will be penetrating him. You will "own him," however temporarily, and he should get the maximum pleasure out of this new experience. This is erotic. It's sexy. Help him embrace it. Pay attention to the subtle and not so subtle emotions he's experiencing and remember one of my core principles about sexual fulfillment:

> *It's not what you can do to him;*
> *it's where you can take him.*

How To Use 'Frottage' To Heighten His Receptivity.

Let's get back to bringing him to a fever pitch. Again, it's important to amplify his desire for your dick to be inside his body. The best way to do that is to give him a simulated experience that does not require him to worry about the pain. For example, let's say you're on top of him and you slowly part his thighs with your knee. Take his hand and put it on your erection so that he can feel the strength and power of your manhood. As he's doing that, slowly place your dick between his legs so that he can feel the heat and the hardness on and around his anus and perineum. Slide it in and out, and back and forth in an undulating motion. This is technically known as "frottage"–a sexual rubbing or 'non-penetrative sex.' It's used to induce sexual pleasure by applying your body to someone else's. You can really see this play out, in of all things, music concerts and nightclubs (moshing's appeal lies in rubbing bodies, not just carrying, jumping or throwing people).

Play with different frottage angles and positions, making sure that you occasionally put his hand on your erection to heighten his desire. This will also make you want him even more.

Engage the erotic feedback loop.

Energy requires dialogue not monologue. Amp it up by responding to the things he says or does. If he says, "I want you inside of me" you can say, "I want to start slow and slide it in and out of you so you can feel how hard and long it is." Not only are you creating more energy but you're giving him erotic feedback—knowledge he can use to turn you on in the future.

The erotic feedback loop is an important part of being sexy. You're not just taking turns speaking and doing—you're creating an energy spiral. The more excitement you show the more he'll want to excite you. You say something that turns him on, he responds with something that turns you on and suddenly you're booked on an inter-planetary flight.

Once you've heightened the sexual tension to the point that he's concentrating on pleasure and not fear, his sphincter will be far more receptive. Now is the time to put some lube on your fingers and explore his butt. It's imperative that you start slowly and sensitively. Stroke the surface of the anus slowly, teasingly. Do not just jam your fingers in as if you're going to finger fuck him. That's a great way to make him seize up. Think feather not leather. The softer you touch him the more receptive he's going to be emotionally and the more welcoming he will be physically.

Think of it as making friends with his sphincter. You don't want him to fear you, you want him to like you. To trust you. To know that you mean pleasure not harm.

> The best way to make him more receptive to bottoming is to give him a simulated experience that does not require him to worry about the pain.

Insert your finger in slowly. Did I say slowly? Because I meant S-L-O-W-L-Y. When it comes to your ass, an inch can feel like a foot. Make sure you play with his penis so that he associates the insertion of your finger with pleasure. Again, do not finger fuck him by moving your finger in and out. In fact, once your finger is in don't move it and keep playing with his penis.

Build Sphincter Trust.

Once your finger is in there comfortably, playfully ask him to tighten his sphincter. Stay with me as there is a very specific reason why you're doing this. As he squeezes you're going to feel the pressure on your finger. While you think of how awesome that's going to feel once your penis is in there you are actually, unbeknownst to him, training him how to relax his sphincter. You see, it's not possible to hold your sphincter tightly for very long. And what is the opposite of tight? Loose. What is the opposite of tension? Relaxation.

Do you see where I'm going with this?

Once you've done that a few times insert a second finger in as sensually as you can. Then repeat the sphincter-tightening request. This is going to do two things: First, you are teaching his sphincter that it can expand without any pain and get it used to something bigger than just one finger. Second, you are continuing to teach your partner how to tighten and relax his sphincter. This will serve you well as you advance to inserting your penis.

Keeping His Sphincter Relaxed As You Enter Him With Your Dick.

Are you ready for the moment of truth? This is how it's going to go down (or in as the case may be). You're going to put the head of your erect penis comfortably, but snugly on the outside of his anus. There should be no space between the opening of the sphincter and the head of your penis.

Have you ever been pinned to a gate at a crowded outdoor event? You weren't going to be pushed through it but you couldn't move away from it either. That's the feeling you're aiming for.

Once you've secured that position, ask your partner to clinch his sphincter as tight as he can for as long as he can. He'll be able to do that for about 20 to 30 seconds maximum. You will be able to tell when his sphincter starts to relax by the look on his face but ask him to tell you anyway because you need to time this correctly.

As he begins to relax his sphincter (he will have no choice as it is physically impossible to keep a sphincter tightened for very long) slowly insert your penis into him. Now, notice what just happened: You are entering him at the point that his sphincter is most relaxed. You've used physics and physiology to create an ideal time for penetration.

"Sphincter Muscle Failure" is the key to pain free bottoming. The concept capitalizes on the nature of muscle failure so that you enter him at the moment when he is most relaxed.

Let's Hammer In The Key Concept.

To understand just how well this method works to ease the pain of penetration it'll help to do a few experiments. Launch the stopwatch feature on your smartphone. We're going to time how long you can keep your sphincter clenched.

Ready? Set? Clench! As the stopwatch ticks on I want you to notice a few things. Your clench is strongest in the first 7 to 10 seconds and then begins to attenuate. Around the 20 to 30 second mark you will experience the beginnings of muscle failure. Not much longer after that your sphincter will relax on its own no matter how hard you try to clinch. This is because your sphincter is nothing but a ring of muscle and no muscle can stay contracted forever.

The key concept here is to penetrate him when he is *involuntarily* relaxed. Not when he's *trying* to relax but when he has no choice but to relax.

Now it's true that the sphincter will automatically seize up as something enters it but the beauty of this method is that the muscle failure guarantees the "rebound clench" won't be very strong if it happens at all. To see this physiologic process in action I want you to time another one of your sphincter clenches.

Ready? Set? Clench! Wait for total muscle failure. As you feel your sphincter relax, try to tighten it right away. You will notice one of two things: 1) It is very difficult to tighten it again. 2) If you were able to close it you didn't get it anywhere near as tight as you did when you first began.

To see how this physiologic experiment applies to bottoming try it in the shower. First, tighten your sphincter as hard as you can, then immediately try to insert a finger into it. You'll notice it is practically impossible to do it without causing yourself a lot of pain. This perfectly captures the scenario of trying to top an inexperienced bottom. Now, clench your sphincter until muscle failure. As you involuntarily relax insert your finger. See how easily it went in? And it wasn't even painful was it?

> The key to pain free bottoming is to exploit the
> nature of muscle failure so that you enter him at the
> moment when he is most relaxed.

What About Topical Analgesics Like Anal-Eze?

Topical anesthetics like Anal Eze or Oragel are bad ways to, er, get to the bottom of your problem. Or rather, the problem of trying to bottom.

Why? *Because anything that masks pain is going to cause harm.* Besides, the anesthetics won't work. They don't penetrate far enough to relax the sphincter muscle. It's like using full sentences to seduce a party boy: Good luck.

If your partner really wants to try topical anesthetics you'll need a prescription from a doctor because the over-the-counter crap doesn't work. And if you do manage to get a prescription, I'd love to see your insurer's reaction to the diagnosis. I mean, what's your doctor going to say to get the treatment approved? "Patient has trouble getting fucked in the ass?"

Topical agents like Anal Zee have some unintended consequences even for porn stars, which is why most of them don't use it. As one porn star bottom told us:

> *I was shooting a film for a weekend period, and the first night I had gotten ripped up by a top and I had to compensate for that by using a numbing cream like Oragel or something similar. But anyhow, I used it numb my ass so I could keep on shooting that weekend and one of the tops (another top) was playing with my ass and was beating my hole with his cock and got some of the Oragel on it and it went soft because my "ass cream" numbed his cock. So when he pulled out, his dick was soft and numb. The whole thing was, the giggle was, that my ass was so tight that it had made his dick go numb.*

What About Poppers?

There's a lot to be said for poppers, but there's a lot to be said against them, too. Let's start from the top. What are poppers? They're a liquid made from the alkyl nitrite family. Most commonly it's slang for amyl nitrate (AM-il NYE-trite), but it's also known as amyl, butyl, and isobutyl nitrite. In prescription form it's used by inhalation to relieve the pain of angina attacks. It works by relaxing blood vessels and increasing the supply of blood and oxygen to the heart. There was a popping sound when you crushed the cloth-covered glass capsules they used to come in, hence the darling name.

"Poppers" as a recreational drug are illegal, but they're sold legally by a sleight of hand—they're marketed as air fresheners, video head cleaners, leather cleaners or even nail polish remover. You'll also see them referred to as 'aromas,' 'liquid incense' and by brand names like Liquid Gold and Rush.

How Poppers Work To Loosen Your Sphincter.

Right before intercourse, the bottom partner sniffs the fumes in a bottle of poppers. Within seconds, chemicals in the fumes cause blood vessels to dilate, which drops blood pressure and increases heart rate. There's a rush of blood to the head, your heart beats fast and all your muscles relax. Especially, the sphincter muscles. Most people who use poppers feel an excited, light-headed feeling for 1-2 minutes before the effects wear off.

People use poppers because they work. They really will loosen your sphincter. They'll also lower your inhibitions.

But like all drugs, the downsides are enormous and you'd be a fool not to consider them.

Poppers Can Interfere With Erections.

Poppers are a perfect example of the law of unintended consequences. Yes, they loosen the sphincter but they relax *all* muscles in the body. Including the muscles that support erections. One of the main side effects of poppers is impotence. In fact, when porn star bottoms want another sniff of the poppers during anal sex, the top often has to turn away so he doesn't breathe in the fumes and lose his erection.

I'm guessing your partner is not looking to lose his hard-on when he bottoms, so that's a giant red flag if you're considering using poppers. Now, not everybody loses their erection but enough do to warrant a good hard think before you use them.

Do Poppers Cause HIV?

Absolutely not, but studies show they might play a big role in getting HIV passed on if you're not conscious of how they can affect your body and most importantly, your behavior. Examples:

- Poppers expand blood vessels everywhere, including the lining of your rectum, increasing the chances that you'll bleed.

- Poppers can affect your judgment, leaving your senses, as well as the unused condom, on the floor.

- Because poppers really do relax the sphincter, you might be tempted to have rough sex, which increases the chance of internal bleeding.

- Poppers temporarily make the immune system weaker, leaving you more open to infection.

Do the math. Increased chance of internal bleeding + cloudy judgment leading to no condom/rough sex + weaker immune system = High likelihood of HIV transmission. If you ask an HIV expert to describe the most likely scenario of an infection, it would go something like this: "When an HIV negative man uses poppers while bottoming for an HIV positive guy who doesn't use condoms."

But Wait, There's More Bad News.
What, that's not enough? Hey, don't confuse the message with the messenger. There are a few other things you should know about poppers. The most common side effects are headaches and dizziness (sometimes immediately). Some people faint, which makes sense because poppers dramatically lower blood pressure. It's the main reason you should NEVER use poppers if you're taking Viagra, Cialis or Levitra. All of these drugs lower blood pressure. Combining them is a great way to risk death.

Poppers aren't addictive but they can be habit-forming. Plus, the more you use them the less effect they have, so you have to keep sniffing more and more to get the same effect.

Should You Use Poppers?

I'm not your mother. Or your doctor. It's up to you. I just want to make sure you have all the facts before making a decision. Under the right conditions they might make sense for you. People are people and there's bound to be curiosity about doing what so many porn stars do to bottom without pain, so as a public service I want to introduce you to...

The Intelligent Way Of Using Poppers.

In the spirit of making sure that curiosity doesn't kill the cat, I've outlined the safest way for you to use poppers. Let me be clear, I am not advising you to use poppers. I am advising that if YOU decide to use them, that you put some thought into how. I spoke to several drug experts and here's what they consider an intelligent approach to using poppers:

- Do not use poppers if you take drugs or supplements that lower blood pressure. This is especially true of erectile dysfunction drugs like Viagra or supplements like Yohimbe.

- Do not use poppers if you have low or high blood pressure, a heart condition or glaucoma or are using medications to treat these conditions.

- Do not use poppers if you're using other recreational drugs like ecstasy, speed, cocaine or crystal meth. They all put strain on your heart.

- Only sniff the fumes. Keep the liquid in the bottle. You will get a chemical burn on your skin if you spill it. It's easy to spill it with lubed up fingers, so be careful! Wash off with water if you do spill it. God help you if you get it in your eyes. Call 911 immediately.

- Never, ever swallow the chemicals in the bottle.

- Keep poppers away from cigarettes, candles and lighters. They are extremely flammable.

- Avoid forcing air into a stuffed nose. The chemicals can cause ear and sinus infections.

- Use the dose doctors recommend for their angina patients: Pass it back and forth close to your nose and inhale the vapor several (1-6) times.

- Use the repeat dosage strategy doctors recommend for their angina patients: Repeat within 1-5 minutes. Do not exceed a total of 2 doses in a 10-minute period. Again, for the intellectually feeble, let me repeat that. ***Do not exceed a total of 2 doses in a 10-minute period.***

CHAPTER FOUR

Combining The Best Position With
The Most Pain-Free Angle Of Entry.

Missionary? Doggie-Style? Straight in?
Angled Up? It Matters.

When I talk about the best position and angle of entry I don't mean the best for you. I mean best for your partner. That's because the most delicate time during intercourse is initial penetration. If you don't find a position that will eliminate the pain or at least significantly decrease it to a tolerable level, the only bottom you're going to see is the ass-end of a liquor bottle.

So the initial penetration is all about him, not you. In fact, I want to introduce you to a very Zen concept—in order to be in charge, you have to relinquish control. In bed, that means the bottom, the submissive guy, is in control (at least initially). Here's why: pain-free bottoming requires *the bottom partner* to find the best position to straighten out his S curve, estimate the best angle of entry and control the pace of it. How is he going to do that if you take control?

The only way he's going to avoid pain and experience pleasure is to control the way your penis goes in and out of you. And in and out. And did I mention in and out? I know that relinquishing control might seem a bit of an irony—isn't bottoming about surrendering yourself to another man? How can you surrender when you're in control? Isn't that an oxymoron, like "jumbo shrimp" or "pretty ugly?" Not to get all Zen up on your grill, but "controlling your surrender" is one of those contradictions that defy explanation. It cannot be explained but it can be experienced, as you're about to find out.

The top is never in charge. At least not at first.

Once your partner has enough experience with bottoming, he can begin to loosen the controls and be "taken" in a way that adds to the blissful experience of surrender, but for now, know this: The top is never in charge. Listen to one famous porn star top:

"In my personal experience it's best for the bottom to take charge. I usually penetrate them only with the head of my dick and have them hold onto my leg or hip and they would be the one to pull me more inside and a little bit more. If I'm too deep, pull me out. I work at their pace."

For once, I can tell you unequivocally, LISTEN TO PORN STARS. If your partner wants to experience pain-free bottoming he has to take control. And the best way to do that is to review our understanding of the puborectal sling.

Sling Forth & Multiply.

Remember, everyone has a puborectal "sling" that surrounds the rectum and pulls it forward toward the navel causing it to have an S shape. Your rectum is not vertically shaped. It's shaped more like an s-hook.

This is important to know because an object entering the rectum at the wrong angle runs into the rectal wall of the first part of the S curve. And that will make you feel like a bat is beating your insides. Let's repeat our previous experiment but this time with a twist: hold your left hand up as if you're shaking hands. This is your rectal wall. Now take your right index finger and poke the middle of the palm at ninety degrees. This is the penis stabbing the rectal wall. Watch it, that hurts! Now, angle your palm (to the left) to 45 degrees and poke again. Better, but it still hurts, right? Now, raise your right finger up by a few degrees and poke. Ahh, feels nice, right? Notice the finger slides up the "rectal wall" rather than poking and jabbing at it. You are not stabbing the rectal wall because you "straightened out the S curve" (your palm) and adjusted the penis' angle of entry (your index finger).

You've just learned two important lessons about topping: Straightening the S curve and adjusting the angle of the penis' entry will eliminate all your partner's pain. Now, how do you adjust his S curve and what angle should you guide the penis toward? Let's investigate.

The Secret To Straightening Your S Curve.

There is only one thing that will straighten your partner's S curve: The position of his legs in relation to his torso. The closer his legs are to his torso, the more his S curve will straighten. His S is at its "curviest" when he's standing up or laying down with heels touching the ground. It's at its straightest when his knees are pulled up close to his chest or shoulders. Any position that creates at least a ninety-degree angle (doggie style for example) will do a lot to straighten his S curve. No position will completely straighten it, though, so you will have to make adjustments by trying different angles of entry.

The S curve varies from person to person. Some have very little curve so almost any position straightens it. Others have a curve so pronounced they have to put their feet to their ears to straighten it, and even then it won't do much. Some people's S curves have different shapes and lay in slightly different locations within the puborectal region. It's almost impossible to say which position will straighten the S curve for your partner—and make bottoming more pleasurable—because it's a function of his anatomy. The only way you're going to find out is to experiment. Different positions (missionary, doggie style) may or may not sufficiently straighten out his S curve, but there is *one* that will absolutely maximize it. And this brings us to…

The Best Position For Pain-Free Bottoming.

Lying on your back and having your partner squat onto your

penis straightens out the S curve better than any single position. Millions of men try bottoming on their back, on their knees, on their stomachs and God knows what other positions, only to stop because it hurts too much. But the minute they try squatting onto an erect penis, everything changes. Why? Let's do an experiment. Get in the shower (don't take this book with you—it isn't waterproof!), lube up a finger and draw in your finger. Notice there's a certain difficulty? Now, squat all the way to the ground and do the same thing. Notice how much easier the finger got drawn in? Amazing, isn't it? Squatting loosens the puborectal sling, allowing the rectum to straighten out so that it comes close to being vertical. The conclusion is obvious: It is far easier to draw an object into your rectum when your knees are closest to your chest. And which position draws the knees closest to your chest? Squatting.

Of course, there are some disadvantages to the squatting position. There's a certain awkwardness associated with bottoming for the first time (as there is for anything) and squatting opens up your body to visual inspection in ways that being underneath your partner does not. It can make you feel exposed and vulnerable. There is also a sense of separation from your partner because your torsos, especially

> Squatting loosens the puborectal sling, straightening the rectum so that it comes close to being vertical and allowing pain-free passage of an erect penis.

the heart area, aren't touching. Some people need to feel the heat of their partner's body to feel more secure.

Still, having your partner experience a few moments of awkwardness is a small price to pay for being able to insert your penis easily and without pain. Squatting gives him more control than any other position. It completely avoids the clumsiness of you poking your penis in different parts of his butt because you can't quite find his anus (it's the gay version of playing Pin the Tail on the Donkey). It also eliminates the possibility of you thrusting in hard and painfully.

Once you're inside of your partner it doesn't take much to roll over (with your penis inside him) to get in different positions. Of course, you don't have to start by squatting. Pick any position he feels comfortable with.

While squatting straightens out the S curve better than any other position, it does not straighten it out completely. Although you've significantly reduced the risk, you still run the danger of your penis stabbing your partner's rectal wall. You can solve this problem by understanding...

The Best Angle Of Entry.
Remember your finger poking your left palm at ninety degrees? When you "straightened the S curve" in your palm, it made it easier for the finger to move forward, although not completely. But when you raised the angle of the finger? Magic! It slid along the "rectal wall" of your palm easily and

without resistance. The lesson: Your partner—*not you*—must guide your penis in so that it slides along the rectal wall rather than poke at it. Your partner is the only one who can do this effectively. Only he intuitively knows what path your penis should take. Only he can immediately course-correct at the hint of discomfort. Only he can do all of this at a pace that's comfortable for him. You? I say this with love, but what you don't know about his S curve is a lot.

It's difficult to say which angle of entry is right for him because so much depends on things that are unknowable— where his S curve begins, how straightened it becomes in certain positions, the natural angle of your penis (does it curve? Left or right? How much?) and more. However, all things being even the best angle of entry is:

About 15 degrees *away* from his navel.

Why? Because the puborectal slings forces the first curve in the rectum *toward* the navel, exposing more "perpendicularity" of the rectal wall to the entering penis. By guiding the head of the penis away from the navel (but not too much!) the penis will be more parallel to the rectal walls. This will avoid the stabbing sensation beginners feel.

Get back in the shower and do this: Squat and draw your finger in toward the navel. You'll notice how quickly you hit the rectal wall. If you keep pressing up you'll hit the prostate (yeah, that's the sensitive jab you just felt). Imagine what it'll feel with a penis going in that angle. Ouch! Now, pull your finger out (slowly!) and draw in your finger, this time completely away from the navel. Notice you didn't really feel any "stab?" That's because your finger lies parallel to the back of the rectal wall when it's fully inserted. Obviously, you don't want your penis aiming for the back of the rectal wall (you would have to stretch your penis backward). I just wanted to show you the dramatic difference between angling the penis toward and away from the navel.

Your partner—*not you*—must guide your penis in so that it slides along the rectal wall rather than poke at it. And always about 15 degrees away from his navel.

So, again, the best angle of entry is about 15 degrees away from his navel. Now, there is something you should be aware of…

The Right Angle + A Straightened S Curve Is Not Enough To Avoid Pain.

Inserting an object into your rectum naturally tenses all the muscles surrounding the rectum. Even a penis going in at the right angle in a straightened S curve will hurt if the surrounding muscles tense up and clamp down. In fact, the tension and constriction will tighten the sling and bring the curve back to the S shape with the penis still in the rectum. Can you say "OUCH!?"

Now, you can't consciously relax the S curve but you can give it the opportunity to—by proceeding s-l-o-w-l-y. Going slow gives the muscles in the puborectal region a chance to relax and re-interpret the insertion of the penis from "Attack!" to "Ooh, pizza delivery!"

By the way, all anal and rectal muscles clamp down in response to fear, stress, and anxiety—in or out of bed. When you describe an uptight guy as a "tight ass," you aren't just commenting on his personality.

Okay, back to you: Go slow and give your partner's rectal muscles a chance to get acclimated so they re-interpret the presence of your penis favorably and relax on their own. Remember this about the nature of involuntary muscles in the rectum: You can't force them to relax. You have to let them let go.

Once You're In, Then What?

Why are you asking me? You should be asking him. Does he need you to stay still? Does he want you to begin thrusting? How deeply? Does he only want shallow thrusts? Ask him. Does he want to change positions? Try it. Does he want to masturbate? There is no right or wrong; only what feels good and what doesn't.

Remember, he's only in control during the initial stage. If you sense that he's okay (because he said so or he looks so), stop asking him questions. Get ready for your close-up because you're about to take over the show.

CHAPTER FIVE

How To Get The Most Pleasure
Out Of Being Inside Him

Speed, Depth & Thrusting Techniques

My mom always said, "You've got to preheat the oven before you stick in the turkey." What a wise woman, my mom. You need to listen to her. While some guys who bottom like the "grab it and growl" school of packing, forcing and stuffing, they are in the extreme minority. You are much better off *gradually* working your way to full penetration and then *gradually* speeding it up.

Here's why going slow is so important: It creates a sense of safety, both from an emotional and physical standpoint. In order for the tissues, muscles, s-sling and sphincters in the puborectal area to relax and become aroused they need to feel safe. The faster and more forceful you go the more your partner's body is going to clench down. Slow, careful movements will support a sense of safety for him and set the stage for deeper levels of arousal.

Never Thrust The First Few Moments Of Penetration.
Once you're in you've got to give your partner's body time

to adjust. The anal canal is extremely adaptable—it can expand enough to accommodate the size and width of an erect penis, but this can only happen slowly. Did I say *slowly*? Because I meant S-L-O-W-L-Y. If you start thrusting right away you're going to seriously hurt your partner and create a whole lot of mistrust that might shut the whole scene down.

Once you're in, FREEZE. Stay exactly where you are. Enjoy the tight, wet sensation as his body acclimatizes to its new expansion. Now is the time to kiss him (if you haven't already been) and do a body language check. Is he writhing in pain? Breathing fast? Squinching his eyes as if he were just impaled by a fence post? Or does he seem like he's got some discomfort but ready to move forward? Once you top a lot you can sense what he needs simply by observing his reactions. But it never hurts to simply ask, "How are you doing?" Believe me, he'll tell you.

> Pain is searing and sharp. Discomfort is a dull pressure. Pain is something to avoid; discomfort is something to accept— because it's fleeting and a pathway to bottoming pleasure.

If you've entered him correctly—amped up his pre-penetration desire so that he's more receptive to your hard penis and used the sphincter muscle failure technique so that you penetrated him when his sphincter was at its most relaxed—

he should be at different levels of discomfort, but no real pain.

Understanding the difference between pain and discomfort can help avoid injury and develop a peak sexual experience. Pain is searing and sharp. Discomfort is more of a dull pressure. Pain is a signal that something is wrong. Discomfort is a signal that you're feeling something unfamiliar. Pain is something to avoid; discomfort is something to accept. Why? Because once you get used to discomfort it goes away and gets replaced with pleasure. Not so with pain. Enduring discomfort will open up new sexual vistas. Enduring pain will open up new rooms at the ER.

If he's in pain ask him if he wants you to pull out. If he's not, ask him if you can thrust slowly. Or simply do it without asking *but only after sensing he's okay.* Let's talk about asking your partner questions for a moment. There is a thin line between showing concern and showing insecurities. If you don't ask enough questions it'll look like you don't care about him, but if you ask too many you'll come across as too solicitous, insecure and in some ways overbearing. That's why it's important to sense what is going on with him and act accordingly. If you see somebody who's hot and sweaty do you really need to ask him if he wants a glass of water? Why don't you simply hand one to him?

Sex is about sensing and responding; it's not about verbally checking in every 5 minutes. At any rate, let's assume that he's not in pain and he's ready for you to start moving in and out of him. What's next?

Let's Talk About Thrusts.

Thrusts are rhythmic in-and-out movements that increase sensation for both partners. Great lovers have learned that it isn't just about in and out, and in and out and did I mention, in and out. Whole new dimensions of pleasure can be added to lovemaking by being creative with thrusting techniques. The best lovers create a dance of churning, deep thrusting, then shallow thrusting, and then reversing the dance. You are trying to take your partner somewhere and the journey will be far more interesting if you show him different views.

A Great Tip

Penetrating him with just the tip of the penis is a wonderful sensation for both of you. This is a great way to start a thrusting pattern, or to occasionally revisit during a love-making encounter. Using just the tip is a way to tease and build arousal, before further penetration or engulfment. You can explore this with slow or quick movements, and everything in between. Try different angles and positions to find out how this feels best for both of you.

Long, Slow, and Deep.

Long, slow, and deep penetration is a great way to slow time, increase arousal and let him feel the entirety of your penis. It's also a great way for you to feel the snugness of his ass from base to glans. After having gradually worked your way to full penetration, take some time just enjoying the lusciousness of the entire penis moving in and out. Going slow can also create some unusually intimate moments with your partner, especially if you lock eyes as you go in slowly.

Lube Up. And Down And All Around.

When it comes to lube, nothing succeeds like excess. Use a lot of lube before and during anal play. Count on needing a lot of it. The penis penetrating the anus should feel as though it can glide inward and outward, effortlessly and smoothly, without causing any discomfort or pain.

What Speed Should You Use?

There's no one right speed to use for any position on any guy. It all depends on the mood. However, there is one general rule that applies to almost everyone almost all the time. *Always start slowly and gradually build up speed.* How much speed you build up depends on what you and your partner enjoy. Once you understand how different speeds affect your partner's experience you'll be able to figure out which speed is appropriate for each stage of your encounter.

91

Press and hold

Sometimes it's good to use no speed at all. Sometimes it feels great to slide your cock as far into your guy as you can and hold yourself there. As stated earlier this is good to do in the first minute after initially penetrating him because it lets his rectum acclimate to being filled up. But it's also a great technique to use later, especially if you want to introduce a little emotion or romance. There's something about just being in his body, with no movement, that creates an aura of union that thrusting sometimes glosses over.

Gradually Faster & Gradually Slower.

You can spice up a sexual encounter by suddenly and dramatically changing up the speed of your thrusts, but don't use that kind of "Stop/Start" technique too much because frequently changing your thrusting pace is likely to throw off your partner's rhythm. Remember, you're doing a dance, and if you don't give your partner some kind of signal of where you're going you're liable to er, step on his feet.

There is one general rule that applies to almost everyone in almost all situations: *Start slowly and gradually build up speed.*

Your partner isn't going to be an innocent bystander in the proceedings. If he's any good (God willing) he will dance with you, not just simply be your receptacle. He'll dip to the left to accommodate your dip to the right. He'll meet the oncoming penis with an incoming pelvis. But if you suddenly and furiously change speed, depth and technique you will throw him off and you'll end up wondering why you had no chemistry in bed.

It's okay to go slow for a bit and then speed it up as long as it's not jolting. Fluidity and flow are your goals, not any pre-conceived notions of the "right" speed or depth. Sometimes guys want their butts caressed like delicate flowers, and sometimes they want to be fucked into the mattress so hard the bed breaks and the snooping neighbors light a cigarette. Both of those techniques are valid. The art is in finding the appropriate time to use them.

Medium Thrusting
After fucking him slowly for a few minutes, his mind and body will be ready and hungry for harder, faster thrusts. Chances are, you will be too. Fast thrusts are great, but don't underestimate the value of medium-paced thrusts. Your partner will get to experience the full sensation of your penis when you thrust at a medium pace. Sometimes he can lose sensation down there if you thrust too quickly.

Taking It To Pound Town.
Medium-paced thrusting is a good standard speed, but any technique used too often will become boring. When you

start out a sexual encounter going slow, then speed up to a medium pace and then finish fast you cover all your bases. The question is, what percentage of the time should you go fast? A good rule of thumb is 10-30% of a sexual encounter. Is that a little or a lot? A little, if you're in shape; a lot if you're not. If you start running out of steam but know that you need to take it up a notch, consider making your thrusts harder instead of faster. You'd be surprised how hard of a pounding an ass can take. It gives your partner more of what he wants and leaves the option open for you to go faster later.

Jack Rabbit Fast

Generally speaking, you can give a bottoming guy a more intense orgasm by speeding up your thrusts. Partly it's because his prostate responds better to shallow, faster motions (your penis stimulates it as you go in and out of him). And partly it's because males *generally* like an increase in speed and pressure as they approach orgasm. This is your chance to lose control and fuck him with reckless abandon. Better a raging gladiator than a panting Pomeranian.

Time Out For A Great Question!

Hey, woody!

I'm an average sized guy (almost 6" but not girthy) and I'm interested in a guy that seems to have a preference for bottoming, but that's my problem. I really like those types of guys (slightly fem) but I'm a huge bottom boy too! So, I'm considering switching my preference. Sex isn't the top thing on my list so I could easily go either way if that's what the guy likes. So my question is, how can I please a bottom, having little experience in the topping department, and while having an average-to-small sized cock? I honestly don't mind the size of my cock—it's proportional to me (short/skinny) but I've had a few guys mock me about my size. It may have been playful but it still sinks in after a while because they were serious. I just want to know if the size of my cock is going to affect my ability to top (well) and what I can do to combat that. I've topped a couple guys in the past and had no negative reaction, but I want to learn to do it right with the equipment that I have.

—Topsy Turvy

Dear Topsy:

The next time somebody says something about your dick, call them out. Like, "STOP. You've got a couple of body parts that aren't so great but I respect you enough not to say anything negative. I'd like the same respect."

Now, about this ridiculous idea that you can only top well if your name is Tripod: The facts don't support you. According to condom manufacturers, only 6% of men need extra large condoms. Are you saying the other 94% are lousy tops? Puh-leeze.

You actually have an advantage, you know. Versatile guys tend to make better tops. If you know what you like done, you'll know what needs doing. As a top, you're more likely to have extra patience during the entry phase because as a bottom you know an inch feels like a foot. As a top you're more likely to re-apply lube because as a bottom you know that nothing succeeds like excess.

But enough of the basics, let's fast forward. The thing that separates the men from the hens is the thrust. And here's a big, wide open secret: ALWAYS vary your thrusting patterns.

The law of diminishing returns says pleasure is inversely related to repetition. You know how the first few bites of a steak always taste better than the last few? It's because you didn't pause, take a sip of wine, or a bite of a side dish. Taste buds get sensitized easily. So do manginas. So, mix it up with these classic Tantric thrusting patterns:

The "Thrusts Of The Heron": Deep for three consecutive thrusts, then go shallow. Think of it as crime prevention: Three strikes and you're out.

The "Thrusts Of The Dragon": Nine times deep, one time shallow. Then reverse.

The "Thrusts Of The Phoenix": Run a pattern —9 deep/1 shallow, 8 deep/2 shallow, 7 deep/3 shallow, and so on until you reverse it and get to 1 deep/9 shallow. Hey, it's the new math.

The Mouse: Quick and shallow thrusts.

The Eagle: Hold your penis motionless at the entrance of his starfish then swoop in quickly and deeply. Like your frenemies do when they see you talking to a hot guy.

These are general rules. Remember, different thrusts for different butts. Variety ain't just an industry magazine; it's a spice of life.

Hit It Like Elvis.

Pumping your penis into him like the head of an oil drill is a good way to hit him deep, hard and fast, but it can feel impersonal and miss a lot of sexual nerve endings inside and outside the anus.

You can hit more nerve endings and add another level of interaction and intimacy to the missionary position by gyrating your hips like Elvis. Think what your pelvis looks like when you swing a hula-hoop around you. Using your hips rather than just the weight of your body changes the trajectory of your penis. Throughout the course of a single thrust your penis hits the anal walls from different angles. There's not an exact science to gyrating your hips during sex. Just make sure they're fluid. Remember, fluid and flow are your touchstones.

Using your hips takes a lot of muscles and is difficult to do with a lot of force or for a long time. It's best suited during the slow-to-medium paced stages of sex when you're warming your partner up.

> You can hit more nerve endings and add more pleasure if you thrust not with your whole body weight but by gyrating your hips like Elvis.

What Not To Do When You're Pounding Him.

While tastes and preferences can vary widely between guys there are definitely some universal no-go's. Among them:

Pulling out completely. It can pack air inside your partner's bum which can lead to "fuck farts," embarrassing all parties to no end.

Putting your weight on your partner. Your partner will find nothing erotic about his inability to breathe. Yes, be on top of him, but use your knees, arms and feet to make sure you're not dropping the entirety of your weight on him.

Not warning your partner before you climax. First, you're missing a great opportunity to build up anticipation. Second, your partner might want to climax with you. Remember I said sex is a dance. Always signal your next move so you don't step on your partner's feet.

Staying quiet. Sex fires on all five cylinders when you verbalize your internal state through words, moans and groans. Eliminating one of those cylinders is going to diminish the pleasure of your encounter.

Changing The Thrusting Pattern When He's Close To Coming.
Whatever you're doing the instant you sense that he's going to come is what you should be doing until he completely ejaculates. Now is not the time to try a different position or change the depth or speed of your thrusts. The reason is simple: Never interrupt momentum. Ever notice that during masturbation

you don't change your stroking pattern as you near the point of no return? You might grip it with more pressure and increase the speed but you don't fundamentally change the stroke, say from tight and fast to loose and slow. The same applies while you're topping him. If he's going to blow while you're pumping him slow and deep, continue pumping him slow and deep. Do not fundamentally change your thrusting pattern.

Coming Before Your Partner Does. Generally speaking, nothing will be more disappointing to the bottom partner than a top who comes first. You'll have to pull out and that means he has to ejaculate *after* you cut his pleasure in half. It's also bad for you as a top. You *want* your partner to ejaculate with your hardness inside him because once he attaches the pleasure of an orgasm to bottoming he will want you again and again!

What You're Aiming For: His Prostate.

A great deal of the pleasure you get from bottoming comes from the penis stimulating the prostate as it thrusts in and out of the rectum. Let's talk a little more about the prostate, which many people call, "The male G-Spot." The prostate is a walnut-sized gland located between the bladder and the penis (just in front of the rectum). It produces fluid that nourishes and protects sperm. During orgasm it squeezes this fluid into the urethra where it mixes with sperm and comes out as that whitish semen many of us think of as the nectar of the Gods. In fact, the prostate produces almost all of your semen.

Obviously, the prostate is crucial to your experience of orgasm. You know that moment of "ejaculatory inevitability" when you're about to come and you feel it deep inside you before anything comes out? That's because orgasm starts with the contractions of the internal sex organs (vas deferens, seminal vesicles and the prostate). Therefore, stimulating the prostate in just the right way can create enormous sexual excitement. In some men, simply stroking the prostate can make them spontaneously orgasm. But the truth is, prostate stimulation is not a universal pleasure and it accounts for a great deal of the reason that some men don't like bottoming even when it's pain-free.

If you want to maximize your partner's pleasure you have to stimulate his prostate in just the right way. Let's take a tour of you own prostate so you can get a better understanding of how to stimulate his. Wash your hands, get undressed and pull out the lube. I'll wait. And for God's sakes, close the curtains!

Ok, ready? Let's rock.

Step 1: Gently Press Your Middle Finger Against Your Anus.

Lay on your back, spread your legs and press your lubed-up

middle finger against the anal opening (you can use the index finger if you prefer, but the middle finger gives you more reach). *Make sure your hand is in the palm up position* (palm pointed to the ceiling). And for the love of God, do it s-l-o-w-l-y.

Step 2: Gently Probe The Anal Wall Upwards Towards Your Navel.

The prostate is located behind the anal wall in the direction of your belly button (two to four inches from the sphincter). Be careful! The prostate is very sensitive. Do not poke and prod. Caress and stroke. Press gently. Use feather-light touches. You're looking for a walnut-sized fleshy ball hiding behind the anal wall. Finding it is a little like playing hide-and-seek, only you're using your finger rather than your eyes.

Step 3: Find And Trace The Contours Of The Prostate.

Once you locate it, trace your finger around the gland. Take a tour. Notice where it is. Make a mental note of how far in (and up) you had to go so you understand the general location of where it will be inside your partner. Ask yourself how stroking your prostate feels. Good, bad? Pleasurable? Ambivalent? Don't judge; notice.

Can't find your prostate or not sure if you have?
The easiest way to find your prostate is to make sure you're sexually aroused. Your penis isn't the only

thing that gets full and erect when you get excited—so does the prostate. So much so that it bulges into the anal wall, making it very easy to find. During arousal the prostate fills with semen fluid. The closer you get to orgasm the firmer the prostate becomes and the easier it is to find and stroke.

You can also try different positions. For example, some guys have better luck laying on their left side and putting their right hand behind their back while bending the knee of the top leg.

Step 4: Massage The Prostate.

You need to exert firm pressure without pushing too hard. Firm but comfortable is your goal. Start at the top of the prostate and slowly push down toward the center. Then go back up. Then start at the bottom and slowly push upwards toward the center. Experiment with different directions to get different sensations. There's no right or wrong way to find out what you like. Be curious and try anything as long as you do it slowly, with care. The prostate actually has two lobes. If you can detect each lobe you can take turns massaging them. Don't be surprised if a couple of drops of fluid come out of your penis, even if it's not erect. This is what many doctors do to "milk" the prostate and relieve pressure in patients with enlarged prostates.

Step 5: Massage The Prostate While You Masturbate.

You may or may not have had an erection while exploring the prostate. It's now time to purposefully get one. Massage the prostate as you masturbate to climax. It is quite eye opening to feel your prostate enlarge as you're about to orgasm and then feel the entire rectum—sphincters and all —rhythmically contracting as you ejaculate. Use this experience to guide your next topping session.

You can also try a more indirect route to stimulating your prostate—finding the pressure point on the perineum directly below the prostate. Do this: Put your index and middle fingers together and gently press the fingertips on the area between your anus and the scrotum. Southerners call this area, "The Tain't" because it "tain't your ass and it tain't your balls."

Start at the boundary of your sphincter and *gently* press up. Move an 1/8 of an inch toward your scrotum and press up. Keep going and you will eventually find the sweet spot— generally, it's the most sensitive spot in a most sensitive area.

Stellar Tip!

You can wring the last bit of semen out of your ejaculation by doing the following: Right after you ejaculate, press your fingers upward starting at the edge of your sphincter and glide them firmly (but gently) toward the scrotum. As you reach the scrotum, clasp the base of your penis and squeeze up to the head. You are basically squeezing the last bit of toothpaste out of the tube—start at the base (the area just above your sphincter) and keep squeezing until you reach the opening (the tip of the urethra). You'll see extra semen come out that you didn't know you had in you. If you're a "dripper" after you ejaculate (you continue to drip semen even after your penis goes soft) this will completely eliminate it.

Was It Good For You?

Some guys find prostate stimulation unbelievably pleasurable while other guys find it extremely annoying. Some men only like it after a certain point of sexual arousal while others like it at any time. Still others don't care for it at all. Individuals vary widely. What causes ecstasy for some causes boredom in others.

It doesn't matter whether you like prostate stimulation or not. What matters is that you experience the process. It is quite astounding to feel your prostate thicken and grow inside the anal wall as you get closer to orgasm. It will give you a fascinating glimpse into your sexual response and a sense of respect for the process your body goes through to deliver pleasure. It will also give you insight as to what's happening to your partner when you're one topping him, or hell, even if you're giving him a hand job!

All Thrusting Aside...

So far we've only talked about the mechanics of topping because without them you are guaranteed to have less than a stellar experience. But it's important to remember why you're taking this journey in the first place. This is not a science experiment and you are not a lab rat. You are topping for very specific, human reasons: You want to feel closer to your partner; you want to give him something of yourself. You want him to feel the presence of your essence inside him. You want to dominate him. You want him to submit to you. You want to *give* him mind-numbing pleasure. You want to *get* mind-numbing pleasure. He's loved your cock in his hands and in his mouth and now he wants it inside of him. You want to feel the kind of physical, sexual union that can only come from giving yourself fully to him.

It's important that you ignite your sexual imagination, stay present to the beauty of your partner's body and enjoy the psychological and emotional journey that penetrating offers.

The Secret to Being Good in Bed.

Think back to the most memorable sex you've ever had. What do you remember most—that thing he did with his tongue or the feeling of getting sucked into a vortex of sexual energy that made you temporarily forget your name?

Being good in bed isn't just about technique. It isn't about what you can do to him; it's about where you can take him. Technique isn't unimportant; it's just insufficient. Getting good at the mechanics makes you a skilled worker. Understanding how to shape passion into a give-and-receive union makes you a sublime lover. So before we dive into techniques, let's paddle around this passion thing.

Passion is a funny thing. You can't teach it because it's not a skill. You can't acquire it because it's not a possession. And you can't learn it because there are no instructions. Like the wind, you can't see it but you can feel it.

> Being good at technique just makes you a skilled worker. Generating passion—now *that* makes you a sublime lover.

While I can't "teach" you passion, you can learn how to set the stage for you to express it in your own unique way. If passion has one defining characteristic, it's energy. Movement. Action. Convergence.

By movement I don't mean sexual calisthenics—setting up a trapeze, swinging from the chandeliers, and diving into pillowed mosh pits. There's nothing wrong with that, but passion defines movement as something that builds and resolves anticipation. Movement that creates the unexpected. Movement that travels from dissonance to harmony. It can be subtle, silent, or loud. It can make you shiver, sigh, or scream. It can pull you down like a whirlpool, suck you up like a tornado, or waft you aloft on a magic carpet. Consider the passionate kiss:

He stops an inch before your lips. The space between crackles with anticipation. He doesn't back up. He doesn't move forward. You're caught in his tease. Your heart climbs the stairs. He leans in. Your lips part and…

This is sexual energy in motion: It holds a chord and waits for the resolving note. It pushes you to the brink and pulls you back just in time to push you again. It has an upward trajectory, transferring from one partner to the other. Movement is passion's starting point. It can be subtle (an unresolved kiss) or explicit (throwing each other around like rag dolls).

Let's do an experiment. Think your worst thought—I don't know, something like going home alone on a Saturday night. Got it? Okay, now really concentrate on that thought as you follow my directions: Rub your hands together as fast as you can for ten seconds. Notice the tingling sensation when you stop? That's movement creating energy, which manifests as heat. Now where did that awful thought of yours go? Poof! Movement creates energy that makes thoughts disappear.

Now, with passion as the backdrop, let's get back to skills. Being good in bed doesn't mean knowing every position in the Kama Sutra. It's combining sexual energy (movements characteristic of passion) with pleasure-giving skills. Remember, bedroom competence creates more desire for you, your body, and of course, your penis. Your goal is to get so good at sex that the laziest guy on earth would take one look at you and say, "*You make me want to get a job.*"

CHAPTER SIX

How To Get Harder Than Algebra

Solutions To Performance Anxiety, Condom-Induced Impotence
& More

Unfortunately, there are several things about topping that can turn Willie into Will Not. They range from performance anxiety to a dislike of condoms to simple fatigue (topping is a lot of work and if you're not in shape it will have an effect on your erection).

The simplest and most effective way of getting and staying hard is to concentrate on what turns you on. With everything that goes on during intercourse that can sometimes be more challenging than it appears. It's easy to get distracted by internal thoughts that don't serve you.

For instance, you may be worried about his hygiene, or where you put the lube, or whether you should use a condom. Or whether or not you can stay hard with a condom given that last week you didn't. You can also be distracted by your insecurities. Is your penis long enough? Is it wide enough? Can he see your protruding belly from this angle? Is he going to judge if you don't do it right?

There are lots of thoughts they can soften your hardest intentions but they will have no effect if you simply remember the golden rule of hard-ons: Concentrate and act on the things that turn you on.

What does that mean? Visually and physically cultivating your personal brand of desire. This is harder than it may appear. Many people don't know what they want. Some are so fearful of expressing sexual desire their subconscious blocks them from conscious awareness. For example, if you come from a culture with strong codes about what males are expected to do (topping) then you're probably going to have a hard time admitting you want to bottom.

You will not get your hardest hard-on if you're too shy to specifically request an act, a position or a technique that turns you on. And it's not enough to ask for what you want. You must also state how you want it.

And even when you do know what you want—and have no hang-ups about it—you often don't communicate it. And when you do, there is often a lack of specificity. Let's say you love getting head. There are two levels of communication you should be engaged in: 1) Telling your partner what you want and 2) Telling your partner *how* you want it. Some people do a good job of #1 but suck at #2.

Part of the hesitation of making a highly specific request ("I

really like it when you look up at me as you give me head")
may be a lack of understanding of what makes you feel
good. And part of it may be that you're too shy or afraid
he'll react negatively. Either way, it's easy to remain at a
lower level of horniness (and hardness) because you do not
know or are too hesitant to communicate what turns you
on.

Erections Love Communication.

What's the answer? Be aware of what you like and move
towards it, physically, emotionally and verbally. For example,
if biceps turn you on and you don't state it, or put yourself
in a position where you can see or touch his arms, it will
have a negative effect on your erection. If you're too shy to
specifically request an act, a position or a technique that
turns you on, you will not get as hard as you can. If you
don't create an environment in which your erection can
come to full presentation you're asking for trouble.

Performance Anxiety.

As Masters and Johnson, the great sexologists, put it, "Fear
of inadequacy is the greatest known deterrent to effective
sexual functioning." Truer words were never spoken.

The problem is in the term itself: "Performance anxiety." A
lot of us think of sex as an act, a performance, with roles
we're expected to play—especially as a top. Much of our
anxiety around sex comes from societal expectations of

masculinity (you're always horny, always hard) and watching porn (you're big as a bridge, never go soft and cum like a waterfall).

Men typically view sex as goal-oriented, performance-driven, orgasm-centric and erection focused. It's great to get hard and ejaculate but when that's seen as the only acceptable form of intimacy it works against the nature of sex as pleasure shared between two people.

Studies show that about one-third of men experience some type "situational impotence" *at least once a year*.

By the way, you're not alone if you happen to have a couple of episodes where you couldn't get as hard as you wanted. Studies show that about one-third of men experience some type "situational impotence" *at least once a year*. In other words, over the course of their lives almost 100% of men will experience "situational impotence" (defined as not getting hard enough or staying hard enough for intercourse). For gay men, these are the typical fears:

- You won't get hard enough

- Your dick isn't big enough

- You will disappoint your partner

- Your partner will compare you to other guys

114

- Your partner will judge you and tell the world

- You'll ejaculate too soon

- You'll take forever to ejaculate

These anxieties produce stress hormones like cortisol, adrenaline, epinephrine and norepinephrine, which produce a heightened state of alert. It's the opposite of feeling relaxed and calm and in the moment, which is necessary for proper sexual functioning.

These stress hormones constrict blood vessels, inhibiting blood flow, which makes erections more difficult. They also increase muscular and body tension, and actually desensitize the genitalia. Be clear that not getting hard enough for penetration doesn't cause that—it's your worry and anxieties about it that do.

How To Deal With Performance Anxiety

Again, the key to getting hard and staying that way is to move your consciousness, your environment and your actions toward a positive flow of desire. Ask for what you like. Touch what you want. Take what you need. All day long we try to rein Willie in. It's time to let him run the show. If you find yourself in a negative loop because you've had a couple of disappointing moments, or if you're just obsessing about the possibility of failure there are a few things guaranteed to put you back in the saddle:

Make A Distinction Between What You Can And Can't Control.

You don't have control over a sexual disappointment but you do have the choice not to catastrophize it. You can choose to stop exaggerating the importance of your perceived failure or shrink the importance of what went right. You can choose to appreciate the pleasure you received before or after the perceived failure.

Keep It In Perspective.

It is what it is. Keep your opinion out of it. Didn't get hard enough? It means nothing but that in that instant you didn't get hard enough. Don't "therefore it." As in, you didn't get hard enough, THEREFORE you're a failure or THEREFORE you'll never get hard again.

Polarized thinking is when a person thinks in extreme terms with no middle ground. Filtering is when you pick out a negative and dwell on it while discounting the positives. Be aware of these terms so you can label your thoughts and have some power of them. For example, if you start ruminating that this "always happens to you" you can stop yourself and say, "Whoa! Hold on, that's polarized thinking. Am I really prepared to say 'always?' What about all those other times everything worked fine?"

If a session didn't, ahem, rise to your expectation the

reaction should be, "Oh, well but everything else sure was hot!" You should walk away intact if you have a negative experience. Don't turn an attempt at sexual satisfaction into a source of grief. It is what is —a mild disappointment, not an earth-shattering event like a murder or a tsunami. The bigger problem you make it the bigger problem it becomes.

Set Realistic Expectations.

You are a man not a machine. You are fallible. We often disappoint ourselves and others but those disappointments don't define us. It's not realistic to think that every sexual experience is going to light the heavens and part the waters. It's realistic to expect a wide variety of sexual experiences—including some awful ones. Experiencing sexual difficulties is the price of being human. You should actually expect sexual failures once in a while because that way you won't be so shocked that yes, you too are human.

Learn More About Sex.

Sometimes guys have performance anxiety because they're inexperienced with sex so they're walking around with wrong information and making false assumptions. Read more books. Learn new techniques. Educate yourself. Check out my two favorite sex books—*Anal Health & Pleasure* by Jack Morin and *Hot Monogamy* by Patricia Love. Oh, and of course, don't forget my other book, *How To Bottom Like A Porn Star*!

Know That Porn Doesn't Qualify As Sex Education.

It's hot but its value is in entertainment, not education. In porn, everyone has a big dick, stays hard for hours and comes like the Trevi Fountain. It's pure fantasy and not anything you should compare yourself to.

What Should You Do At The Exact Moment You Can't Get Hard Enough To Penetrate?

It's one thing to fear something that hasn't happened or to judge it after it does. But what do you do in the moment? Suppose you're about to enter him and for whatever reason you go soft?

Internally, I want you to think the following: "Oh yeah, there's that human thing again. It's okay it's only temporary." And then I want you to remember that during sex the penis is constantly going up and down. Sometimes mysteriously. For example, have you ever had a raging hard on, gave your partner head and noticed that although you were turned on during the whole act your penis actually got much softer? *This is perfectly normal.*

So let's get back to the no-big-deal moment where you went soft (or not hard enough to penetrate). State the obvious to your partner. Say something like "Oh, I'm not hard enough right now" and get off him. If you went soft because of a distraction (the phone rang, the dog barked) or because there's a physical problem that can be corrected (a bad position that cramps your leg), then correct the distraction and get back to business.

If it's simply because you had an inexplicable "moment" then get off him and concentrate on other sexual pleasures (oral, manual). Sometimes you just need a different kind of stimulation to be at your hardest. Should you attempt to top him if you get hard again? No, if you feel like you have to prove something because that's a recipe for a repeat. Yes, if you can't wait to get inside him. But the bigger answer is that it doesn't matter. It's just not that big of a deal in the scheme of your sex life if in that particular moment you top him or not.

Another highly effective method to get your groove back is to engage in "Pattern Interruption." That means temporarily taking a break from the activities. Go to the bathroom, get something to drink or turn some music on. The point is to "reset" your body by interrupting the current path or pattern. You'll be amazed at how a five or 10-minute interruption can clear the deck for your dick.

Keeping It Hard For The Condom.

There you are with a raging hard-on (boy, you get a lot of those, don't you?) But the second the condom goes on you go limp. You get more and more upset about it, which only makes matters worse. Are you alone in this? Does this happen to others? What can you do to keep an erection with a condom on?

I'm not going to sugar coat this: Condoms are awful. Only vaginas have the power to elicit more gay impotence. We hate them (condoms, not vaginas, although you could make a case for them too) for good reason—their awful texture, their medical smell and that wonderful power they have to reduce sensations. Condoms suck! But HIV and other STDs suck even more so we're stuck with the suck. Still, there are ways of making peace with them before they rip your erections to pieces.

Improve Your Environment.
There you are, kissing, hugging, with his legs around you ready to be plowed like a snowy Minnesota highway. Your whole body is pounding with pleasure and anticipation when suddenly you have to switch from passion to logic. Where are the condoms? Are they in the first or second drawer? And where's the lube? Do you have enough of it? You stretch to look under the bed and, of course, it's not there, so now you have to get up to look for it. Ah! There it is! Now look down. Your dick just went from impressive to impossible. Losing your erection is natural when your attention goes from the throbbing excitement of sex to the logical pursuit of safe sex.

Solution: Be prepared. Always keep lube and condoms near the bed. Best bet: Keep a "fun box" near or under your bed so you ALWAYS know where everything is—and always within arm's reach. Remember, Preparation = Penetration.

Shake Hands With The Devil.

How often do you use condoms? Let's pretend you use them every time you top somebody (ha!). But how often is that? Unless you have bottoms throwing themselves at you or you're a sex addict who'd fuck a snake if you could pry its bottom open, you're probably not having a lot of intercourse. That means your only experience with condoms is what, once every couple of weeks? Once a couple of months?

Not only do you have relatively infrequent exposure to condoms you only reach for them at your most vulnerable moment—naked, hard and in a hurry. That is a recipe for condom-induced impotence.

Here's a better idea: Buy buckets of condoms and spend 20 minutes a day for a few days, opening them, stretching them to the breaking point, and noticing the different smells and textures. Do silly things with them like filling them with water, tying their ends and playing catch with them. Why? To desensitize yourself. To take their power away. By the time it's 'showtime' you won't be intimidated because the look, texture and smell of the rat bastards will be so familiar.

Get knowledgeable.

Do you open a condom from top to bottom? Side to side? And then once you've gotten them open, which side do you put on the head of your dick so you can roll it down? Confusion is another great recipe to scare the hard off your on.

Solution: When you're alone, get yourself "excited" and put dozens of different condoms on. Notice they're like socks—there's a right side and a wrong side. How do you know the difference? The "Teat." Make sure you put it on with the teat pointing upward. Also, practice opening them quickly and carefully.

Stellar Tip!

Stick with an easy-to-open brand. For instance, my favorite brand has a slight "V" cut that makes it obvious where to tear it. A lot of condoms don't have instructions or "clues" like a "V" cut, and you can literally try tearing the four corners of the square before you find the right entry point.

The main thing is to become intimately familiar with condoms BEFORE you have sex. That way you'll have power over them rather than the other way around.

Why Tops Need Condoms.

The second most common way of getting HIV is to be the top in rubberless sex. True, the risk isn't anywhere near being the bottom in unprotected sex, but it's still pretty risky. Some respected scientists put the chances of catching HIV at 1 in 50 if you're bottoming and 1 in 500 if you're topping (without a condom). But the truth is no one really knows. And trust me, you don't want to be the guinea pig who finds out.

So here's why tops are at risk if they don't put the jacket on:

1. During the excitement of sex, what with all the endorphins and adrenalin rushing around, you're less likely to feel micro-abrasions or scrapes on your dick.

2. There is almost always blood inside a man's hole, even in bottoms who've fucked so much they have an odometer in their anus. That's because tearing often happens during sex. And don't forget, 75% of all men, gay or straight, will have hemorrhoids. Don't be fooled by the fact you can't see the blood—sometimes they're invisible specks that never leave the anal canal.

3. Whatever's inside a butt (blood, fecal matter) is going to go inside your "piss slit" and into your urethra, which is lined with soft mucous membranes that tear easily. As you back out to thrust again, the urethra closes, pushing down the "material" that just entered further down the shaft, scraping and scratching it. Lovely thought, isn't it?

Now, do the math: 1+2+3=HIV.

Do Guys With Big Dicks Have More Trouble With Erections?

Most urologists don't report a connection between big dicks and a rougher time getting a full erection. However, researchers believe it may be easier to treat erectile dysfunction in men with shorter dicks.

Because so many treatments rely on partially increasing blood flow to the penis, they believe treatment for erectile dysfunction is more effective in men with smaller dicks (because they require less blood to fill them up).

Too Pooped To Pop?

Most guys who've never topped before are quite surprised by the strength and stamina it takes to get the job done right. The truth is, if you're not in relatively good shape you're not going to be a very good top. That's because you're basically doing all the work and that includes some heavy lifting, holding, grabbing, setting up, scooping, buoying, elevating, raising, moving, and of course, humping.

And I'm not even talking about an especially acrobatic session, either. Even in a short encounter *you* have to take control, *you* have to be the one to set the positions, the angles, and the leverage. And that takes strength and stamina. I suppose you could lay there like a wilted piece of lettuce and let him climb on top of you cowboy style, but that just makes you a lazy top and a miserable lover.

There's a fair amount of stress on your knees when you're humping and you can work up a good sweat if you get a good rhythm going. All of that is going to impact your erection if you're not in shape. The solution is obvious: Get in better shape. Exercise not only improves blood flow to the penis but the conditioning will help you keep it up longer.

A Word About Alcohol.

Winston Churchill proudly said he'd taken more out of alcohol than it had taken out of him. He clearly wasn't in the bedroom when he said it. Alcohol dulls the nerves that transmit sensations. It ups the desire but lowers the performance. It can give you "Beer Sex." Meaning, the hardest thing you'll have to offer your partner is the bottle you're drinking out of.

Alcohol is not an aphrodisiac, but you'd be a fool not to recognize its power to melt away reservations, inhibitions and worries—the three pillars of awful sex. So yes, alcohol can be quite helpful *in moderation*. But what's moderation? Here's how to make sure the bottle doesn't throttle your sex life:

> After about 3.5 drinks, the average 150 lb. man will have erection trouble.

Sip, don't gulp. The liver metabolizes half an ounce of alcohol per hour (about the size of a regular drink). The faster you drink the higher the blood alcohol concentration.

Eat when you drink. Food can slow down the absorption rate by up to 50%.

Phase out the Fizz. Carbonated drinks speed up alcohol absorption so stay away from fizzy mixers.

Hose it Down. Drink a glass of water for every alcoholic drink you take. Alcohol dehydrates, which helps desensitize nerve endings. Water replenishes and flushes the toxins out.

One of the biggest drawbacks to drinking is that after a while it makes you think safe sex is a padded headboard. So the trick is to limit your drinking. But how much is too much? About 3 1/2 drinks for a 150-pound man. Much after that, the only thing that'll be standing upright in your house is the vacuum cleaner.

Are You A Two-Pump Chump?

Premature ejaculation is the most common sexual dysfunction in men under 40. About 30% of men complain about it. Men have subconsciously trained themselves into ejaculating prematurely. As boys we learned to masturbate quickly. (After all, how long can you stay in the bathroom with your mom banging on the door screaming, *WHAT ARE YOU DOING IN THERE??!!!*)

But before you label yourself a Three Stroke Bloke, know that the average session of intercourse lasts about 5 minutes. So even if your partner uses your sessions as an egg timer you're halfway to average. One condom manufacturer said they only need to test their product for 50 thrusts. Doesn't say much for male stamina, does it? Still, the question remains: How quick is too quick? How do you define premature ejaculation? Easy. It's the inability to consciously control or choose when to climax.

If you're a premature ejaculator, don't distract yourself in bed. The problem isn't that you're paying too much attention to your body; it's that you're not paying enough.

Most guys try to solve the problem by distracting themselves —counting backwards from 100, or picturing turn-offs— like dead cats, bank statements, that sort of thing. You couldn't pick a worse a worse strategy. The problem isn't that you're paying too much attention to your body; it's that you're not paying enough.

The first step in overcoming premature ejaculation is identifying and avoiding the point of "ejaculatory inevitability." Or in plain English, "the point of no return." That's when your heave is going to ho and nothing can stop it.

If you're like most premature ejaculators, you're not aware of the subtle cues leading to your orgasms. Fortunately, the "Stop/Start/Change" method will take of that. With it, you can transform yourself from a two-pump chump to a long-time champ. Here's how:

Stop/Start Alone. When you're alone, masturbate until you get close to the "point of no return," then STOP. Do nothing but focus on the sensation of your penis. The urge to orgasm will subside within 3 minutes. Start masturbating again. Do this over and over and you'll find you'll last longer and longer. When you've got that down, go to step two.

Pace Alone. Now masturbate until you get close to coming and instead of stopping, slow down. CHANGE. Change the speed of your stroke, the pressure you put on it and the site of your grip. Take your hand away from the head where there's more sensation to the shaft where there's less.

Stop/Start Together. Have your partner masturbate you until you get close to ejaculatory inevitability then have him STOP. Basically, follow step 1 only your partner's doing the work and you're doing the refereeing.

Pace Together. Now have your partner masturbate you until you get close to coming and instead of stopping, CHANGE. Basically, follow step 2.

Intercourse On Your Back. Lie flat on your back with your partner sitting on top. Do NOT use the missionary position because it uses your muscles differently and it's harder to get relaxed. Insert your erect penis into him. Don't move. Get acclimatized for as long as it takes, taking in the moist, warm pleasure. Now use the stop/start/change method. *You* move up and down. Getting close? Stop. Wait a few minutes. Now have *her* move up and down. Close? Change.

Intercourse In The Missionary Position. Enter him when you're on top. Start moving. S-l-o-w-l-y. Keep using the Stop/Start/Change method throughout. If your partner is any good, he'll pretend it hurts —that way you'll feel like you've got a big one.

Delay Away?

Never use creams or ointments that claim they'll help you last longer. They don't work and you'll end up rubbing it off on your partner, causing him a loss of sensation. On top of that, he may be allergic to its active ingredient—benzocaine (it's a topical anesthetic used to treat canker sores). Think he'll forgive you for taking him to the emergency room when all he wanted was to be taken, period? France doesn't grow enough roses to get you out of that one.

CHAPTER SEVEN

How To Stop Worrying That
Your Penis Isn't Big Enough.

Journal Of Sex Medicine Survey:
Penis Size Stats For White, Black & Hispanic Men

Overheard in the locker-room:

"Would you wear shoes if you had no feet?"
"No."
"Then why are you wearing underwear?"

Gay men are far more obsessed with penis size than straight women are, even though both are sexually turned on by male genitalia. In most surveys women don't even rank it in the top five. So if it generally doesn't matter to women, why does it matter so much to gay men?

First, because we have a bigger is better mentality. I call it Male Math: Size + Size = Status on Stilts. That's why men love bigger cars, bigger biceps, bigger guns, bigger wallets, bigger everything.

Second, gay men watch a lot of porn, where every penis is a kidney-wiping, liver-lifting jabber. So they have a completely unrealistic view of what a "normal" sized erect penis looks like.

> Porn gives you a completely unrealistic view of what a "normal" sized erect penis looks like because they only hire well-endowed performers.

Penile size can be measured in a lot of ways. Obviously, the differences will impact the results. There are two widely recognized ways of measuring your one true thing. The most common is the "You Wish" method popularized by gay dating and hookup apps. It involves looking at your pinky and seeing a thigh.

I'll talk about the second way in a second. First, the bad news: the average penis size is not six inches. The "six inch myth" got started when Kinsey did his landmark penis size study back in the 50's. Although there were 2,000 men in his study, it had a fatal flaw—the results were self-reported. Men were asked to go into a room, get themselves hard and measure themselves. Now tell me, would you believe anything coming out of a man's mouth while he's holding his dick?

Men always lie about size. Why do you think we came up with maps that associate an inch with a mile? Realizing that too many men were backdating their stock options, urologists developed a new way of measuring the size of the prize: A third party. So, now every legitimate penis study includes medical staff doing the measuring and reporting. And guess what happened? The average erect penis size shrank from Kinsey's 6.2 inches to 5.1-5.8 inches, depending on the study.

The Journal Of Sex Medicine's Latest Penis Size Study. Read it and weep: The average erect penis size is less than six inches, according to the latest penis size study in the Journal Of Sex Medicine. And African-American men don't have bigger penises than white men. Combine that with data from the Centers Of Disease Control (CDC) and I have some very bad news for the Blacks-As-Tripods stereotype: Black men aren't bigger than white men in *any* department—not height, not weight, not BMI, and sadly, not penis size.

Hey, what's that sound? Reality cock-blocking another myth. Take a look at some of the eye-opening penis size stats from the Journal Of Sex Medicine and height/weight figures from the CDC:

Size Category	Black Men	White Men	Hispanic Men
Mean Length of Penis (in inches)	5.77	5.58	5.57
Mean circumference (in inches)	4.83	4.82	4.89
Height	5'8"	5'8"	5'6"
Weight	189 lbs.	193 lbs.	177 lbs.
BMI	27.1	27.1	28.0

Please note: The difference in length and circumference between the races is statistically insignificant. This study is relatively consistent with the results of prior surveys.

I may be whispering against the roar of the ocean when I say this, but try to hear it anyway: The totality of sexual pleasure has very little to do with size. Reducing men to a hash mark on a ruler is one of those ignorant, hurtful conceits that gets in the way of great sex.

Sadly, urologists are faced with the dilemma of men with normal-sized dicks wanting penile augmentation surgery because their sense of inadequacy is as big as the lies we tell ourselves. I say leave the urologists alone, for Pete's sake. They have *real* problems to attend to.

> According to the Journal of Sex Medicine's latest survey, the average erect penis size is *below* 6 inches. And black men aren't more endowed than white men.

The average erect penis size is *below* 6 inches. So all you six-inchers who thought you were carrying pellet-shooting nibblets can sigh with relief now that you've gone from "normal" to "LARGE" just by opening this book. You can feel relieved, but you've missed the point. Size has nothing to do with greater sexual satisfaction.

Exactly How Big Are You? Let's Find Out.

The single best way to manage penis size anxiety is to actually measure Willie so that you can deal with facts rather than myths. If you want to know your exact measurements, here is the scientific procedure that urologists use:

1. **Get undressed in room temperature.** "Shrinkage" will occur if it's cold. I don't know about you, but I want every millimeter counted.

2. Use a cloth ruler. Tape measures or straightedge rulers don't measure curvatures well.

3. Lie on your back and start where the base of your penis meets your stomach. Do NOT start from the back of your balls. Nobody includes the basement when they quote the height of a skyscraper, so don't include the tip of your ass in quoting yours.

4. Round up to the nearest centimeter, not the nearest foot.

5. Read it and weep. Most men will fall below six inches. Check against the chart above to compare other stats.

Actually, there's a much faster and easier way to measure your cock. You don't even need to get hard to do it. All you have to do is stretch your flaccid flogger and measure it from the penopubic region to the tip. Believe it or not, every major study shows a high correlation between erectile and flaccid/stretched length.

When all is said and done, the majority of us will fall somewhere below six inches. Skip the weepy letters about how awful it is to have an average-sized dick. Studies show there is no, as in none, as in nunca, proof that having a big dick leads to greater sexual satisfaction.

How To Tell If You Need An Extra Large Condom.

Here's an interesting trick I learned from a condom company. If you want to find out if you have a big dick without measuring it, then put a tube of toilet paper over your erect penis. If it slides all the way down to the base, you're average or below average. If it gets stuck, then pop the champagne corks because you're one of the lucky few. Yes, FEW. Condom manufacturers estimate that only 6% of the population needs extra-large rubbers.

Final Thoughts.

If you follow the instructions in this book you will be able to top like a stud. This might make you want to top the entire western world but I'd like to offer a cautionary tale against doing it with inappropriate people. Meet my friend, Doctor Dave. He could never top until he read this book. He wanted to try his newfound skill on multiple partners but he worked 14-hour days at his practice, so he didn't have the opportunity to meet a lot of people. Unfortunately, he ended up having sex with several of his patients. He tried to rationalize his behavior by reminding me that he was single, that his patients were single, that he wasn't the first doctor to sleep with his patients and that nobody was harmed by the experiences. Finally, he asked for my advice.

I said, "Dave, *you're a vet.*"

My point, and I do have one, is a) never take your pets to Dr. Dave, and b) don't take sex so seriously. No matter how serious sex gets, there's always room for laughter. Thank you for allowing me to help you experience a better sex life. Now, go. Top like a stud. And don't forget to laugh.

About The Author.

I started my career as an op-ed columnist for *Southern Voice*, a gay newspaper in Atlanta. Upset that I won the city's Most Loved Columnist three times in a row, I rallied when I also won the Most Hated category. The editor then approached me about writing an irreverent sex advice column. I thought, "Awesome! Send me your cutest employees and I'll get started!" We syndicated the column all over the country and I sort of became known as the "East Coast Dan Savage." I then went on to write my first gay sex book, *Men Are Pigs But We Love Bacon* (Kensington).

My proudest achievement came a few years ago when I helped create a website that helps parents come to terms with their children's sexual orientation. We get thousands of emails a year from parents and their gay children thanking us for making it possible for them to reunite as a family. If you or someone you love is going through drama and strife about being gay, please visit us at www.familyacceptance.com. Oh, wait, back to my bio! Soon I was writing gay themed pieces for *Newsweek, The New York Times*, salon.com and other publications. I also became a frequent commentator for National Public Radio's All Things Considered. That led to a major production company in London asking me if I'd like to audition for a co-hosting role in a heterosexual sex makeover series called *The Sex Inspectors* (they thought it'd be cool to put the gay in it). With the screen test cameras rolling, I remember the production chief asking me what I thought of women faking their orgasms. "That's nothing," I sniffed. "Men fake whole relationships."

I got the job.

The show went on to be an international hit, airing in 12 countries, including the U.S. on HBO. It led to my biggest book yet, *Sex Inspectors Master Class: How To Have An Amazing Sex Life* (Penguin).

Once during filming, I sat on the bed with a woman I was advising (don't worry, we were fully clothed—it wasn't that kind of show!). The video cameras that we put throughout her house showed how cruelly she rejected her husband's advances. I said, "Put your arm around me, I want to show you how you reject your husband." I whacked her arm away like it was an unwanted fly and looked away from her. Indignantly, she said, "I do NOT do that!" I said, "Yes, you do." She knew I was right. I could see her face softening. I leaned in. "Can I tell you a secret?" She nodded. I cupped my hand around her ear and whispered something. She started bawling. The producer, director and audio people went nuts because the microphone didn't pick up what I said. The director stopped the filming to give the woman time to compose, took me aside and asked, "What the hell did you say to make her cry like that?

I said, "*Men have feelings, too.*"

I love giving advice to people. I love to see barriers crack and humanity come to the surface. I hope I was able to that with the book you're holding in your hands and that you've enjoyed reading it as much as I did writing it.

Check Out My Other Books...

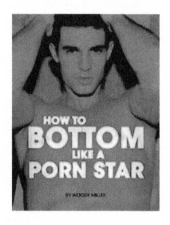

How To Bottom Like A Porn Star

Learn porn star secrets to bottoming without pain and start making love with volcanic pleasure. Written by gay sex advice columnist Woody Miller (me!) and a team of urologists and colo-rectal specialists, this book combines porn industry secrets with innovative techniques from the latest gay male sex research.

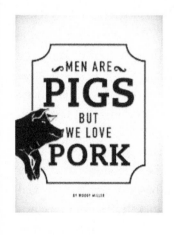

Men Are Pigs But We Love Pork

Gaydatingsuccess.net called it "The funniest collection of gay sex advice columns since Dan Savage!" Sample: On making sure you're clean before doing the deed: "Douche. Gravy's only good on mashed potatoes."

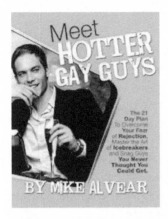

Meet Hotter Gay Guys—

The 21-Day Plan To Overcome Your Fear of Rejection, Master the Art of Icebreakers and Snag Guys You Never Thought You Could Get.

Have more sex, get more dates, or find a husband with this step-by-step manual that shows you how to approach, meet and attract beautiful gay men. From getting rid of fear of rejection to knowing exactly how to start a conversation, this is the ultimate gay dating blueprint.

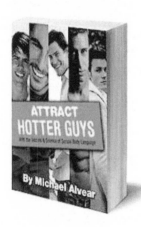

Attract Hotter Guys with the Secrets & Science of Sexual Body Language.

The definitive body language guide for gay men. It's packed with inventive body language strategies proven to make you more appealing and approachable. Learn which gestures, postures and expressions attract gay men—all based on peer-reviewed studies done by leading psychologists in non-verbal communication.

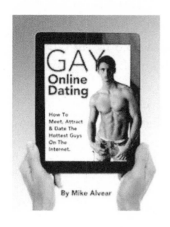

Gay Online Dating: How To Meet, Attract & Date The Hottest Guys On The Internet.

As Manhunt.net's former advice columnist and a consultant for other men seeking men sites, I can tell you exactly what kind of pictures, usernames, head-lines and profiles attract hotter men. I can also tell you why you only seem to attract freaks and flakes. This book is based on focus group research, sur-veys and pattern usage of some of the biggest gay dating sites. Start attracting hotter guys online tonight!

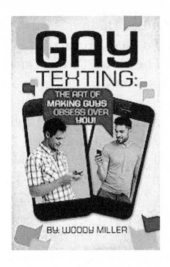

**Don't Get Friend Zoned!
Get Guys To Hang Out Or
Hook Up. Includes...**

- Developing a sense of texting humor that makes guys want to hang out with you.

- "Small talk" texting techniques that get him to respond quickly.

- Turn-around texting tactics that will stop him from friend zoning you.

- How to avoid conversational dead-ends with the concept of "multiple threads."

- A catalog of 300+ witty texts you can send and call your own.

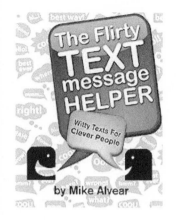

The Flirty Text Message Helper: Witty Texts For Clever People.

A collection of witty texts you can send to your crushes. Hand-picked by our team of writers & researchers, there are no clichés, lame poems or cheesy pickup lines. Categorized by 19 dating circumstances, use these texts to build attraction and score a date. So funny you'll buy it just for the entertainment value alone!

Want More Information On Gay Dating?

Visit my site at grabhim.net and sign up for the free newsletter.

Made in the USA
Las Vegas, NV
06 August 2021

27687191R00090